Healthy
Children,
Healthy Lives

Healthy Children, Healthy Lives

*The Wellness Guide
for Early Childhood Programs*

Sharon Bergen, PhD, and Rachel Robertson, MA

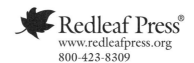

Redleaf Press®
www.redleafpress.org
800-423-8309

Published by Redleaf Press
10 Yorkton Court
St. Paul, MN 55117
www.redleafpress.org

First edition 2013
Cover design by Jim Handrigan
Interior design by 4 Seasons Book Design/Michelle Cook and typeset in ITC Officina Sans Std
   and Adobe Garamond Pro
Photo on page xvii by Carrie Quist
Photos on pages xxiv, 58, 144, and 188 by Steve Wewerka
Photos on pages 8, 36, 68, and 100 by Rachel Robertson
Photo on page 139 by Jennifer Kvidt
Printed in the United States of America
19 18 17 16 15 14 13 12   1 2 3 4 5 6 7 8

Library of Congress Cataloging-in-Publication Data
Bergen, Sharon.
    Healthy children, healthy lives : the wellness guide for early childhood programs / Sharon Bergen, Rachel Robertson.
       p. cm.
    Summary: "Healthy Children, Healthy Lives helps improve the wellness of children, families, and early childhood professionals in early childhood programs. This series of checklists covers six components of wellness-nutrition and healthy eating habits; physical activity and fitness; emotional health and resilience; healthy care practices; safety and risk management; and leadership, management, and administration. Each research-based checklist provides built-in guidance for improvement, complements any high-quality curriculum, and aims to contribute to children's ability to thrive and experience joy in life and learning." — Provided by publisher.
    Includes bibliographical references and index.
    ISBN 978-1-60554-081-8 (pbk.)
    1. Health education—United States. 2. Health education—Curricula—United States. 3. Early childhood education—Curricula—United States. 4. Parent and child—United States. 5. Health promotion—United States. 6. Mental health promotion—United States.   I. Robertson, Rachel. II. Title.
    LB1140.5.H4B47 2012
    372.37—dc23
                          2012024448

Printed on acid-free paper

For my mother, who was always there to encourage her children to be happy, confident, and healthy. Thanks, Mom, for sending me outdoors to play, for reminding me that life's "little things" will come and go, and for making sure my plate was always full of nutritious things to eat. You are the best.

—Sharon

To my children, who put up with the many evenings I spent in front of the computer instead of with them, who tolerated my random food experiments while writing the nutrition chapter—although I may never live down the mashed cauliflower debacle—and who inspire me daily to be someone who tries to make the world just a bit better for them and their generation.

—Rachel

Contents

Acknowledgments

Every book, this one included, ultimately is a team effort. We wish to thank a number of very important members of our team who gave generously of their time and talents and helped to improve this work. First, thanks to the entire team at Redleaf Press. Each of you added a valuable "something" to the book, and it would be a lesser work without your perspective and dedication to the result. We would particularly like to thank the many content experts and reviewers who supported our efforts in developing this book. Some of you provided insight; others reviewed all or parts of the text. For all of these efforts, we are extremely grateful. Your expertise has helped to shape this work, and we acknowledge the value of your input. We hope that we have represented your insights well, and we regret any errors or omissions that may surface. Please know that these are entirely the responsibility of the authors.

We'd also like to thank our families, who have patiently tolerated our absences while we were busily writing this book. They are such avid cheerleaders, they deserve their own pom-poms.

Finally, but most importantly, we wish to acknowledge the many teachers, directors, family child care providers, and other professionals who work so hard to make the world a "well" place for young children. Your responsibilities are many, and we appreciate how dedicated you are to those you serve.

Introduction

For the first time in two centuries, the current generation of children in America may have shorter life expectancies than their parents.
—New York Times, March 17, 2005

Children's health is in jeopardy. In recent years, the number of children who are overweight or obese has skyrocketed, and with this rise has come all sorts of related illnesses and injuries. Children these days are coping with stress, jam-packed schedules, and pressure to perform every day. At the same time, schools and many early childhood programs—even families, frankly—are reducing or eliminating children's opportunities for imagination, play, and physical activity. Our current culture and our daily routines do not support children's healthy development. Worse: our way of life is harming children's health.

Why Early Childhood?

We wrote *Healthy Children, Healthy Lives* because we are alarmed by the health crisis children face these days, a crisis we feel strongly all early childhood professionals need to understand. But equally important, we wrote this book because we believe the community of early childhood professionals can—and must—do something to help.

By taking a complete, proactive approach toward children's health and wellness, we are certain the unhealthy trends affecting children these days can be reversed. We are convinced that the movement to improve young children's health and wellness won't happen in a conference room or congressional session—although organizational programs and a few strategic policies won't hurt. It will happen through the everyday learning experiences a young child has with a committed caregiver. That means you.

Every week over 11 million children in the United States under the age of five spend an average of thirty-six hours in some type of child care setting. During the hours these children are in care, they count on a child care professional like you to meet their health and safety needs and to enable their growth and development. To support these children, caregiving professionals do many things: provide meals and snacks, promote physical activities, guide behavior, offer emotional support, and provide a safe environment in which children can explore. Further, while facilitating the children's growth and learning, caregivers plan and offer experiences that support children's physical and social-emotional health—two domains directly related to a child's overall wellness. In short, child care professionals are tasked with providing for children's overall health and wellness. This is an opportunity we need to capitalize on.

RAPID DEVELOPMENT

Children's early years are the optimal time for influencing their development across their life-spans. During a child's first years of life, development occurs at a rapid pace. Just think about the dramatic physical changes that happen in a child's body between birth and the first day of kindergarten! Children's bodies grow more and faster during these first years than at any other time in their life. Children learn to use their bodies in myriad new ways during this time too—to walk, to talk, to reach, to climb, to run, to build, to write, and so on. As remarkable as this visible development is, the development going on inside children's bodies, especially in their brains, is even more remarkable. Much of the brain's physical development takes place after a child is born. In the first five years, a child's brain forms neural connections that will be used throughout her lifetime.

All the while young children are developing physically, they are also developing socially, emotionally, and cognitively. During the early years, the quality of children's relationships, attachments, and overall social and emotional climate impacts their mental health and cognitive development. Again, consider the differences between an infant and a five-year-old in his ability to express emotions, overcome challenges, and get along with others. While infants have some mechanisms for engaging with others and ensuring that their needs are met, by the age of five, a child has developed many of the social skills she will use throughout her life. She will use these social skills to live and work alongside others and to engage in healthy relationships.

Because all this development—physical, social, emotional, and cognitive—occurs so rapidly in the early childhood years, it is the perfect time to influence behaviors. When very young children start on a path of healthy behaviors early in life, they are more likely to reap the full benefits of their healthy habits. Healthy habits learned early in life have lasting impacts; they become part of the child's lifestyle and natural way of being.

And because development occurs at such a rapid pace in the early years, it is the best time not only to establish healthy habits but also to correct poor ones that have taken root. The longer an unhealthy habit persists, the more challenging it can be to change. Think about your own not-so-healthy habits. Those unhealthy habits that have been part of your lifestyle for a long period can be very challenging to change. Imagine if you would have addressed those habits when they first started, before they became second nature. When you use *Healthy Children, Healthy Lives*, you will promote healthy habits and support children in their development of a healthy lifestyle to last a lifetime.

POSITIVE INFLUENCE

During children's early years, the adults in their lives make a huge impact on their wellness. Very young children are almost completely dependent on adults to protect them from harm and to provide everything they need to grow and develop. Even as children become able to feed themselves and meet some of their own physical needs, they continue to rely on adults to help them make good choices. On their own, children may not choose healthy foods, safe activities, or the other things that support their overall wellness.

In addition, children count on adults to provide good models of healthy habits. As children grow and learn, they take cues from the adults around them. When adults, including caregivers and family members, model healthy habits, children are much more likely to incorporate these habits into their own behaviors.

What Is *Healthy Children, Healthy Lives*?

What is *Healthy Children, Healthy Lives*? It's simple, really. *Healthy Children, Healthy Lives* is a comprehensive resource for early childhood professionals that provides information and guidance on topics related to children's wellness. We use the term *wellness* because *Healthy Children, Healthy Lives* doesn't focus only on the absence of health problems; it also focuses on the presence of good health—both physical and emotional—and preventative practices. For instance, when we discuss physical fitness, we don't just cover ways to ensure children participate in physical activity so they don't become overweight. We also present activities that promote a love of physical activity and the lifelong habits that will help them remain physically active. When children remain physically active during their lifetimes, their bodies and brains function well.

Numerous programs to improve children's health are popping up all over the country, and excellent resources abound: *Caring for Our Children: National Health and Safety Performance Standards; Guidelines for Early Care and Education Programs* addresses children's health issues, such as injury and illness prevention and safety practices. Mrs. Obama's Let's Move! campaign and Sesame Street's Healthy Habits for Life initiative focus on children's nutrition and physical activity. The Strengthening Families Program and the Center on the Social and Emotional Foundations for Early Learning support families and the social and emotional development of young children. We applaud these programs and resources, because it certainly will take more than one voice to improve children's health nationally. We also know how many books and binders sit atop an early childhood professional's shelf and how precious your time is. To make it as easy as possible for you to commit to improving all aspects of young children's wellness, *Healthy Children, Healthy Lives* collects and combines information about and guidance on a broad but pertinent range of wellness topics into just one book. Then it expands on the information and guidance by providing detailed, actionable steps. Through its many checklists and the action plan, *Healthy Children, Healthy Lives* provides a way for you to assess your program's wellness policies and practices and identify immediate and manageable ways to improve them.

SCOPE

There is no doubt about it: *Healthy Children, Healthy Lives* covers a lot of territory, from nutrition education and illness prevention to leadership practices that minimize caregiver stress. Wellness is a big topic, and we believe that addressing it in an all-embracing way is the only way to ensure sustainable results—or, in other words, *to get children healthy!* The scope of *Healthy Children, Healthy Lives* is broad, and it was sometimes challenging to exclude topics we believe are important for children's robust development, topics such as literacy, music, science, and so forth. In the end, we decided to focus on only topics directly related to health and wellness. This means many important topics, especially those primarily related to children's cognitive development, do not fall within the scope of this book.

When choosing a wellness topic, we asked ourselves two questions:

1. Will practices related to this topic improve a young child's overall wellness?

2. Are there simple, actionable steps related to this topic that an early childhood professional can take to make a difference?

Knowing that we answered yes to these questions makes us confident that early childhood professionals using *Healthy Children, Healthy Lives* can make a significant, positive impact on the health, happiness, and even lifespan of the children they care for.

In writing *Healthy Children, Healthy Lives*, we made every effort to delve deeply into a wide range of topics related to children's wellness. But please be aware that the information provided in the book should never be considered a replacement for your child care licensing or other regulators. Programs are encouraged to meet, and even to exceed, licensing requirements as part of the work of providing a healthy environment for young children.

How *Healthy Children, Healthy Lives* Works

Healthy Children, Healthy Lives has been intentionally designed so that early childhood programs and professionals of all types and at any stage of awareness can use it successfully. The book is divided into six parts representing the major areas of children's wellness:

- nutrition and healthy eating habits

- physical activity and fitness

- emotional health and resilience

- physical health

- safety and risk management

- leadership

The breadth of the content included in *Healthy Children, Healthy Lives* represents one of the challenges we share in addressing children's wellness—a great deal goes into providing a healthy program. The good news is that because you are the expert on your program, you get to decide where to start. You get to determine how to use the information provided to best respond to your program's unique needs. For instance, perhaps you're just digging into the topic of children's wellness and want to use the book to assess your entire program. Or perhaps parents in your program are asking about what you're doing to tackle childhood obesity, so you'll use part 1, Nutrition and Healthy Eating Habits, to set program-improvement goals in response to their concerns. Or maybe a third-party adviser or mentor will use the book to help your program qualify for a wellness-related endorsement or grant. No matter, *Healthy Children, Healthy Lives* is a tool that can be used in its entirety, part by part, or even section by section, as need be.

Each of the six parts in *Healthy Children, Healthy Lives* begins by providing an overview of the subject matter and explaining its relevance to early childhood. Each part is then divided into sections that zero in on and describe specific wellness topics, and each wellness topic breaks down into achievable goals and checklists.

Here are the sections, by part, in *Healthy Children, Healthy Lives*:

Part	Section
Part 1: Nutrition and Healthy Eating Habits	Foods and Meals
	Healthy Eating Habits for Infants
	Healthy Eating Habits for Children
	Program Approach to Nutrition
	Nutrition Education and Resources for Families
Part 2: Physical Activity and Fitness	Developing Physical Activity and Fitness Habits in Children
	Program Approach to Physical Activity
	Physical Activity and Fitness Education and Resources for Families
Part 3: Emotional Health and Resilience	Sociability
	Emotional Intelligence
	Positive Behavior Guidance
	Approaches to Learning
	Family Support and Involvement
Part 4: Physical Health	Health Promotion
	Addressing Illness and Special Health Needs of Children
	Environment
	Environmental Health
Part 5: Safety and Risk Management	Safety
	Emergency Preparedness
	Injury Prevention
	Security
Part 6: Leadership	Communicating with Families about Health, Safety, and Fitness
	Leading Program Staff Members
	Facility and Financial Management

CHECKLISTS

You can use the checklists for a variety of purposes: to assess the strengths of your program, to measure growth, to compare administrator and teacher ratings, to establish program objectives, or to communicate with parents and community members. The checklist items—or "indicators," as we call them—represent the ideal, which for many programs will be something to strive for. Just know that improvement will be progressive. For example, the first time you complete a checklist, you may find that your program demonstrates fewer than half of the indicators. Later, after goal setting, action planning, and some effort to improve practices, you may find your program is meeting most or even all of the indicators in the same section. Few, if any, programs will be able to meet all the indicators right away—and that's okay.

Within this book's six parts, there are twenty-four sections; the sections serve to narrow the broad subject matter of each part. Each section contains a few paragraphs explaining its slice of the subject matter, as well as a brief list of the topics covered by the goals and checklists that follow.

Each goal is worded to describe an aspect of an early childhood program's commitment— your program's commitment—to a healthy practice. For example, a goal in the Safety section, under the topic "Supervising Children," is "We plan the environment to optimize supervision of children in our care." This goal statement is followed by a checklist made up of four indicators, which are:

- ❑ The environment is arranged so children are always visible.
- ❑ If our setting has small spaces, closets, or other hard-to-supervise spaces, mirrors are used to help with visual supervision.
- ❑ If infants are cared for, then cribs are kept near the play space. Cribs are not in separate rooms that are unsupervised.
- ❑ Infant monitors or other mechanical devices are never used to supervise children, even sleeping children.

These and all the indicators in *Healthy Children, Healthy Lives* represent the range of ways your program can achieve the goals that facilitate providing a healthy program. The indicators are aligned with national standards, accreditation criteria, current research, and developmentally appropriate practices. The indicators within each checklist are not presented in order of importance or difficulty, because they are all important to the development of a program that fully supports children's wellness. We developed the checklist indicators to be challenging but achievable. Once you dig in, you may discover you're already doing some of the practices described by the indicators. Some practices may even be required by your licensing rules. You may find indicators that describe things you're not currently doing but could do with a bit of effort. You may also find indicators that will be very challenging to achieve, practices that will take a great deal of time and energy to accomplish. All programs will likely find wellness areas where they are already strong and other wellness areas where they have opportunities to improve. Do not expect to check off every indicator immediately, no matter the quality of your program. The purpose of the indicators—of the goals—in this book is to help early childhood programs improve and grow so that children's wellness will improve and continue to improve, now and in the future, and the range of challenge represented by the indicators is intentionally broad.

Some sections also include bonus checklists. Indicators presented in bonus checklists oftentimes highlight innovative, emerging practices and a higher degree of challenge. The bonus indicators describe opportunities for improvement for programs already doing a great deal to meet the related wellness goal. Consider them with a "wouldn't it be nice to do this" outlook and tackle them when the other section indicators have been met.

TERMINOLOGY

Throughout *Healthy Children, Healthy Lives*, we use "teacher" to refer to the adults who work directly with the children—the children's caregivers. We know that in the early childhood field there are a variety of titles used to describe this role, including teacher, caregiver, child care provider, teacher's aide, and floater. In the end, we feel that no matter what your official title is, when you work with young children each day, supporting their growth and development, you are a teacher.

We also use "staff member." When we use it, we mean all employees of the program—bus drivers, cooks, health care professionals, program administrators, curriculum specialists, substitutes, administrators, enrichment teachers, and custodians, as well as teachers. When we use "staff member" in an indicator, the indicator applies to all program employees and not only the teachers. It is important to keep this distinction in mind.

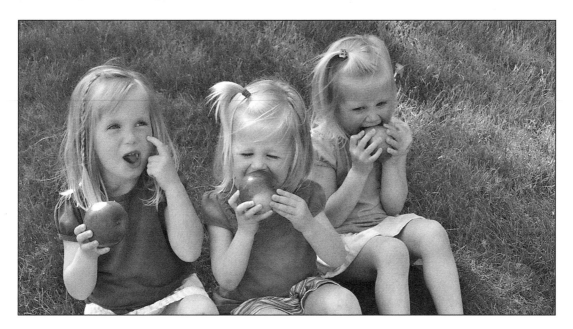

In many indicators, "volunteer" is also used. When we use it, we mean unpaid adults who have contact with the children. For example, your program may have students from a local university who volunteer their time to the program, engaging with the children, to accumulate work experience.

We use "program" throughout the book to represent the wide variety of environments in which children receive care, including family child care homes, center and school-based programs, and community programs. We deliberately use "child care program," "early care and education program," and "early childhood program." We know the early childhood field uses each term broadly, and we want to be inclusive. *Healthy Children, Healthy Lives* is intended for any program serving young children, schoolagers included.

FAMILY CHILD CARE PROVIDERS

We know that some early childhood resources don't feel relevant to family child care (FCC) providers. We don't want this to be true of *Healthy Children, Healthy Lives*. We wrote this book with FCC providers in mind, as well as center and preschool staff members. We understand that the FCC provider is often the teacher, the custodian, the cook, the music teacher, the nurse, and the administrator all rolled into one. If this is true of you, please apply each term we use—teacher, staff member, leader—to your different roles. We are confident that the practices presented in *Healthy Children, Healthy Lives* are just as applicable to and achievable in FCC as they are center-based programs. No matter the type of building or program you work in, it is simply essential that all professionals in the early childhood field understand and prioritize children's health and wellness.

Take Action!

After you select a part or a section or a few sections as your starting point, read through the introductory material. Then you'll be ready to use the checklists to set goals. You may be able to check off some indicators right away, based on what you already know about your program. You may need to observe, ask questions, or find documents to check off other indicators. Your evaluation will provide the greatest value if you consider each indicator thoughtfully and honestly. *Checking off indicators representing practices you hope to do or only do occasionally will not give you an accurate picture of your program.* And without an accurate picture of your program, setting realistic goals and improving practices will be difficult.

Once you have completed the checklists from a section or two, you may feel ready to begin planning some program improvements. First, look at the indicators you did not check off. Are there one or more practices your program could easily add? Or maybe you're interested in working toward something more difficult. Among the unchecked indicators, is there a challenging practice or two you're ready to tackle? Use the *Healthy Children, Healthy Lives* action plan to record your plan of action and to document your work toward the goals you want to achieve.

On the action plan, indicate the part, section, and goal you want to work toward. It is helpful to always keep the goal in mind as you work toward program improvements; the goal often describes both the "what" and "why" of important wellness practices. After listing the part, section, and goal, list the indicator or indicators you want to achieve and the action steps your program will need to take; include the indicators' page number from the book for easy reference.

Next record your action steps. The action steps should break down the program improvement into small, manageable tasks. When you record your action steps, avoid making general statements, such as, "Be more open to breast-feeding." General statements like this one are hard to measure and make it difficult to know when you have achieved the action. Instead, make specific statements, such as, "Create a display featuring breast-feeding information." The more specific the action step, the more clearly you'll be able to measure your progress.

Next identify the resources you will need to accomplish each action step. Resources might be materials such as family letters, program equipment, or food service equipment. Or resources might include the funds needed to make a repair or the people needed to complete a specific task or job.

Once you've identified resources, assign a responsible party to each action step and create a timeline for completing the action. Who will be in charge of completing the task, and how long should it take? The responsible party is the person or the people who will do the work and who will make sure the work gets done. The timeline describes when the work will happen and the date it will be completed. Some tasks will require only a day or two to complete. Other tasks will take longer and have timelines involving months of work.

Finally, identify costs. Some tasks will have no costs. Some tasks will have very minimal costs. And some tasks will be quite expensive and require thoughtful budgeting. Purchasing new furniture for a breast-feeding space could cost hundreds of dollars, but installing and arranging the furniture would have no cost if the work is completed by parent volunteers.

Use the notes column to record your progress. This is particularly important for tasks that have multiple small steps, are complex, or have long timelines. For example, one task involved with creating a space for breast-feeding might be to clean out a small space near the infant room. A first step toward doing this could be to recruit some parent volunteers to take on the cleanup project. When that step is done, use the notes section to indicate that volunteers have been identified, and note the names and contact information of the volunteers. Using this technique, your action plan becomes a one-stop working document for all of your wellness projects.

As you use the action plan more and more, you will become increasingly expert at identifying effective action steps, necessary resources, responsible parties, reasonable deadlines, and costs associated with implementing a variety of checklist indicators. Updating your action plan consistently will help keep you on track. Make notes of the progress you have made. Adjust your timelines as needed when circumstances change. Then, when you complete an action step using the action plan, check it off in the plan's last column: *Success!* When you've completed all of the action steps identified in the plan for an indicator, check off the indicator in the book too. *Another success!* Over time, you will implement your action steps, check off more and more checklist indicators, and achieve the goals you decided to work toward. Remember to celebrate your progress! Each step you take toward improving the wellness practices in your program will make a lifelong difference for the children you care for.

Action Plan

Part: *Nutrition and Healthy Eating Habits*

Section: *Healthy Eating Habits for Infants*

Goal: *We support breast-feeding in our program.*

Indicator/Page Number	Action Steps	Resources	Responsible Party
The program offers new or pregnant mothers reliable information about the benefits of breast-feeding, p. 19	Add a family letter on breast-feeding to infant program folders	Copies of family letter	Assistant director
	Create a display in infant area featuring breast-feeding information	Pictures and information from the CDC website	Infant teacher
The program has a private and comfortable space set aside for mothers to use for breast-feeding or expressing breast milk on-site, p. 19	Clean out small space adjacent to infant room	Solicit volunteers from parent group	Parent volunteers Infant teacher
	Purchase rocking chair, table, lamp, rug, and window curtain	Funds from parent group fundraiser	Director
	Arrange space with new furnishings	NA	Parent volunteers
	Create flyer for families of infants announcing new space	Paper, ribbon cutting supplies	Director

Timeline	Cost	Notes	Success!
Create January 1-15 Add to folders beginning January 15	Cost per page = 3¢ 100 folders = $3.00	Create PDF version for website too	✓
Up by January 15	$15 = copies of photos, display items	Check on supply of laminating film	✓
Recruit volunteers in March Cleanout day April 10	No cost	Contact Mrs. Smith about volunteering Order cookies for volunteers	
Parent fundraiser March 15 Shopping day April 15	$750 (will be raised at fundraiser)	Check out sale at furniture store, bring tax exempt information	
April 16	No cost		
Create flyer April 1-15 Ribbon cutting April 17	$50	Invite health consultant to ribbon cutting	

DEFINING SUCCESS

How you define success is really up to you. When your program has met all—or simply most—of the indicators in a checklist, your program has met the goal. We know some of the goals will be inordinately challenging for particular programs, and some may choose not to implement specific indicators. You do not, after all, need to set your sights on perfection—to achieve 100 percent of the indicators in every section—to continuously improve the overall wellness of the program. Successful programs will make steady progress, tackling new indicators regularly, working toward new goals and the action steps needed to meet those goals routinely.

It will be easier and more rewarding for you, your coworkers, and the children and families served in your program if you celebrate successes as they occur. When you complete a goal or a set of goals, celebrate the accomplishment and give credit to everyone who participated. Highlighting successes as they occur will encourage more and more people to get involved and stay involved. When you've finished creating a private, comfortable space for mothers to use when breast-feeding, hold a ribbon cutting celebration. Thank the parent volunteers who helped to do the work, and call for a round of applause to recognize the infant teacher who volunteered to oversee the project! Take pictures of your celebration and include them in your next newsletter or on your program's website or Facebook page. Volunteers love to be recognized and your appreciation goes a long way toward encouraging them to volunteer for the next project on your action plan.

FAMILIES AND STAFF MEMBERS

Improving the quality of your program by improving your wellness practices will undoubtedly benefit the children in your care. And it's likely you will discover that it also benefits you, your staff members, and the families your program serves. In fact, many practices and policies represented by indicators in *Healthy Children, Healthy Lives* focus directly on improving aspects of staff member or family wellness—which, with few exceptions, will affect the children in a positive way. For example, one indicator in section 13, Family Support and Involvement, reads, "New families are introduced to families in the program. They are encouraged to develop relationships." When new families develop relationships with other families in the program, they build a network of support and resources they can turn to during periods of stress or puzzlement over children's development. Another indicator, this one in section 23, Leading Program Staff Members, says, "Staff members' benefits include paid sick days so staff members are not penalized for illness." When staff members are afforded paid sick days, the children benefit because they are not exposed to illness by their caregivers. Improving your program's wellness practices and policies will benefit so many people.

And that is a good thing because, truly, a child care program administrator will never be able to make sustainable program changes on her own. Engaging families and staff members in the work of implementing *Healthy Children, Healthy Lives* is essential. Create small groups of staff members to help you complete the checklists, identify goals, and create an action plan. Involve parent volunteers by asking them to enact improvements once you have identified them—for example, to install mirrors to aid supervision or to identify sources of locally grown organic food. Engaging families and staff members not only helps to distribute the work of making program improvements, but it also helps inspire families and staff members to become more conscious of their role in supporting children's wellness.

When families and staff members actively support the wellness program, they learn about ways they can evaluate and adapt their wellness practices at home.

So as you set and achieve your goals, you make an important difference for children and their families and for you and your staff members. Although this work will take time and commitment, the benefits will be significant. Most teachers first become engaged in working with young children because they have a desire to make a difference for children. What better way to make a difference than to start a child off on a path toward wellness and healthy development?

ADDITIONAL RESOURCES

We wanted to make it as easy as possible for you to understand and achieve each indicator, so in the book's appendixes, we provided a number of tools to help you implement or improve a practice. If we considered a resource to be essential to your understanding of a related indicator, we included it in the appendix. If we thought a resource would be helpful but not essential to completing an indicator, we provided a bit of information about the resource in the text. The annotated resources in the back of the book also describe a number of resources that, should you access them, will provide more in-depth information on topics addressed only broadly in *Healthy Children, Healthy Lives*. A number of resources and tips for best practices are also provided in sidebars found throughout the checklists.

Healthy Children, Healthy Lives introduces and uses terms from early childhood education and other wellness-related fields. A glossary is included in the back of the book to help you use and understand terms that may be new to you. Terms that are defined in the glossary are presented in the text in bold type.

Without a doubt you will want to celebrate the hard work you do using *Healthy Children, Healthy Lives* to improve children's wellness. To help you promote your accomplishments, we have included a certificate of participation at the back of the book. You can proudly display the certificate to alert families and staff members to your dedication to children's wellness.

To support you in your work to engage and educate staff members and families on the importance of wellness, we also created *Healthy Children, Healthy Lives Training and Resources: Reaching Staff and Families*. This CD-ROM provides you with

- seven complete PowerPoint presentations—one staff training presentation for each of the six parts of the book and one overview presentation of the *Healthy Children, Healthy Lives* program for families and other stakeholders;

- handouts for each PowerPoint presentation;

- fifty-two Info to Go resource flyers for families focusing on a variety of wellness topics; and

- six Info to Go resource flyers for staff members focusing on how the wellness topics relate to their daily work.

In addition, we have developed a Facebook page where we will regularly share tips and strategies, guide relevant discussions, promote best practice sharing, and communicate updates on important policies and initiatives. We know early childhood professionals all over the world have innovative practices and ideas related to children's wellness. We want to ensure that all users of *Healthy Children, Healthy Lives* can interact with, support, and share ideas with one another. To that end, join us at www.facebook.com/HealthyChildrenHealthyLives.

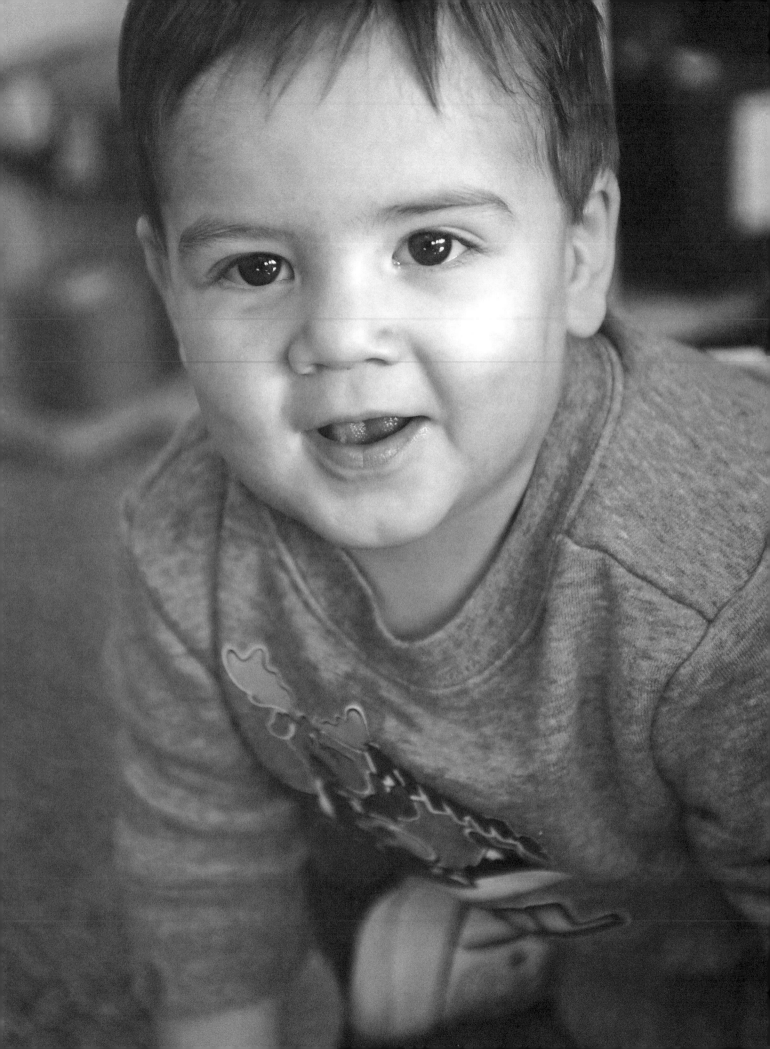

Part 1

Nutrition and Healthy Eating Habits

It turns out the phrase "You are what you eat" is closer to the truth than many of us thought. We now know without a doubt that what we eat has a significant impact on our bodies, now *and* in the future. The foods we choose to eat are powerful; they can positively or negatively affect our overall health, energy level, ability to fight off disease, physical appearance, mental attitude and perspective, and brain development. From pregnancy onward, food and nutrition choices impact a child's life. Many people—including parents, other family members, and teachers—influence a child's eating habits. Being mindful of what children eat can have a substantial impact on weight, physical appearance, behavior, health, and development. So adults tasked with the care and education of young children must be intentional about encouraging **nutritious** food choices and healthy eating habits in children.

Childhood Obesity

Obesity and obesity-related issues have received increasing national attention in recent years, leading to a surge of research and focus on nutrition-related issues. The evidence of our country's obesity epidemic is impossible to ignore. Childhood nutrition and eating habits are in the spotlight because of the alarming statistics that have emerged. Here are some facts:

- Over the past two decades, the prevalence of obesity in children has doubled; at the same time, the number of adolescents who are obese has tripled (AAP 2012).

- Thirty-two percent of children and adolescents are overweight, meaning their **body mass index** (BMI) is at or above the eighty-fifth percentile, and 16.3 percent are obese, with a BMI at or above the ninety-fifth percentile (Cali and Caprio 2008).

- According to Let's Move, approximately one in five children is overweight before age six.

The problem of childhood obesity cannot be solved without focusing on children's nutrition. But childhood obesity isn't the only reason children's nutrition deserves attention from people in the early childhood field. Ensuring that children receive adequate nutrition—for example, vitamins, minerals, and proteins—and adequate amounts of food is equally important. Healthy eating and nutritional support and education must address not only obesity but also **nutritional deficiency** and **food insecurity**.

Nutritional Deficiency

People are considered nutritionally deficient when they do not receive the **nutrients** they need from their daily diets. Nutritional deficiencies occur in children and adults alike. Even those who are overweight can be nutritionally deficient. According to findings from the National Health and Nutrition Examination Survey 1999–2000, 20 percent of the calories consumed in the United States are from **nutritionally void** foods such as soda and pastries (Block 2004). When people subsist primarily on nutritionally void foods, their bodies cannot function properly, and they are more susceptible to illness and injury. Children eat nutritionally void foods for many reasons, including cost, convenience, and access. Compounding the problem is how food choices are made. When children eat typical American "kid foods"—the type of food often found on children's menus in restaurants, such as chicken fingers, macaroni and cheese, and hamburgers—they consume few vitamins and minerals and a lot of unhealthy **simple carbohydrates**. When such foods make up the bulk of children's daily diets, their nutritional needs are not met, their weight increases, their health declines, and their development slows.

Food Insecurity

Not being able to predict when you can eat your next meal or where it will come from is called **food insecurity**. Sadly, hunger remains a significant and disturbing problem in the United States and is a reality for many families with young children. About 17 million children (23 percent of all children in the United States) are food insecure (Nord et al. 2010). For some children, their only regular source of food is eaten while they are in child care. Their teachers must ensure that food for these children is the healthiest possible. As the Food Research and Action Center (FRAC) notes, "The mental and physical changes that accompany inadequate food intakes can have harmful effects on learning, development, productivity, physical and psychological health, and family life" (Why Hunger 2012).

The Link between Nutrition and Learning

Educators should be aware of the strong link between nutrition and learning and academic achievement. Persistent lack of important nutrients in children's diets affects cognitive ability, attention span, ability to concentrate, and IQ. It can also contribute to increased illness and absenteeism, both of which influence children's learning in other ways. Even as seemingly small an act as skipping breakfast or eating a nutritionally void breakfast can negatively affect children's capacity to learn (USDA 1999). If children are hungry or lack needed vitamins, they can't think or concentrate. The education community has a clear investment in the resolution of these challenges and should be involved in solving these problems.

Solutions

Most researchers have found that early prevention and interventions are more effective than adult intervention or education in reducing obesity. Future health challenges can be greatly reduced if healthy nutritional practices are introduced when children are young. Acting on this knowledge, many programs are beginning to focus on nutrition and children's health in new ways. As a nation, we are making progress. For example, in December 2010, President Barack Obama signed the Healthy, Hunger-Free Kids Act of 2010, which increases the quality of foods served in schools. The act also allows a dinner meal to be served to children receiving free or reduced breakfasts and lunches, increases access to healthy drinking water, and eliminates unhealthy choices from school vending machines (WhiteHouse.gov 2010). Farm-to-preschool programs help provide fresh, healthy food to early care and education programs. Weekend backpack initiatives, in which children receiving reduced lunch at school receive backpacks filled with nutritious food to take home over the weekend, are blossoming in communities across the country. Michelle Obama's Let's Move! campaign continues to attract attention and prompt change. But there is still a long way to go.

What Can the Early Care and Education Community Do?

Because children almost always eat meals and/or snacks in early care and education programs, care settings are ideal places to positively influence children's nutrition, food choices, and taste preferences. In their earliest years, children develop attitudes and preferences that become the foundation of their adult opinions and behaviors. Thus, early care and education programs are optimal places for introducing healthy eating habits. This is especially important for the early care and education community, because some research indicates that child care attendance is associated with being overweight (Maher et al. 2008). Supporting children's healthy nutrition and healthy eating habits is multifaceted; it includes:

- being thoughtful about purchased foods,

- ensuring that preparation and serving practices contribute to the overall appeal and nutritional value of the meal,

- ensuring food safety,

- providing an environment that supports and encourages breast-feeding,

- eliminating sugary drinks,

- helping children manage **portions**,

- introducing new foods,

- removing unhealthy food items from the menu, and

- evaluating and changing food-related policies.

These are just some of the numerous ways teachers can make a positive difference that could influence a child for a lifetime.

Of course, families already have opinions and preferences about nutrition. Early childhood education professionals should be cautious not to seem as if they are passing judgment on family choices; instead, they should work together with families to support children's development. All teachers should take their jobs as role models seriously and understand that what they do in front of children and families strongly influences the children. What may seem inconsequential—for example, wrinkling your nose when broccoli is served—can make a lasting impact. Focusing on nutrition should be viewed as a responsibility and an opportunity for everyone in the program. Even adults can benefit from emphasis on nutrition and healthy eating habits. Small changes can bring about big results for all. As a report by Harvard University's Center on the Developing Child emphasizes, "'Getting things right' and establishing strong biological systems in early childhood can help to avoid costly and less effective attempts to 'fix' problems as they emerge later in life" (National Scientific Council on the Developing Child and National Forum on Early Childhood Policy and Programs 2010, 5).

Section 1

Foods and Meals

Nutrition and healthy eating are important concepts for young children to learn. Many of the standards in "Nutrition and Healthy Eating Habits" focus on how to teach and model these valuable concepts. But if the food purchased and prepared in a program does not meet nutritional objectives and guidelines, teaching nutrition and healthy eating won't be effective, no matter how comprehensive efforts in the learning environment are. Thankfully, teachers don't have to be dieticians or chefs to understand these concepts and positively affect children's nutrition.

Food is the fuel for our bodies and medicine to keep us healthy. Rather than choose food just because it looks or tastes good, teachers should choose foods and recipes that help reach health and nutrition goals. This doesn't mean the food can't be delicious; in fact, it should be delicious. It does mean that food choices beginning in early childhood must balance multiple needs and help develop healthy tastes and preferences.

Children must be offered **nutritious** food as often and as early as possible. According to a report by the Harvard University's Center on the Developing Child (2010), "The Foundations of Lifelong Health Are Built in Early Childhood," early learned health-promoting behaviors can influence children's long-term risks for obesity. Many adults can recall what they were fed as children. How many of us have positive or negative food associations that can be traced to our childhoods? If children are offered a variety of nutritious foods when they are first introduced to table food, their taste and texture preferences are positively influenced over the long term. For example, repeated exposure to a variety of whole fresh fruits—rather than sweetened fruits or fruit desserts—is likely to lead to a lifetime of choosing whole fresh fruits. Child care programs that serve fresh fruits and vegetables, lean meats, **whole grains**, and low-fat dairy products are providing valuable **nutrients** for children today as well as building healthy eating habits for life.

Healthy foods do not have to be significantly more expensive or time consuming to prepare than less healthy ones. With proper resources and knowledge, teachers can modify food purchasing and preparation to make them nutritional and cost-effective. Even if high-quality, nutritious foods are slightly more expensive initially, these foods result in healthier, happier children who are better able to learn and develop. In the long run, good food benefits children and programs.

This section will address:

- Food purchasing: Good nutrition begins with the food purchased. Establishing and following best practices for selecting and purchasing foods that contribute to children's nutrition is key.

- Meal and menu planning: Evaluating current menus and adopting effective methods of healthy meal and menu planning is an important part of improving overall program nutrition.

- Food preparation: Practices that ensure food safety, enhance eating experiences, and maximize the nutritional benefit of food are essential components of healthy childhood nutrition.

- Meal and snack service: How meals and snacks are served can impact a child's willingness to try and ability to enjoy new and nutritious foods.

Food Purchasing

When you are ordering ingredients and ready-to-eat food, it is critical to children's health and well-being to make simple and informed choices. Many children's food intake does not meet the USDA's daily recommended nutrient values. Child care programs should make their food purchases purposefully so children get most of the nutrition they need while in child care. Programs can expose children to healthy foods and eating habits while their tastes and habits are still developing by selecting **nutritious** and **nutrient-dense foods** and ingredients.

FOOD-PURCHASING PROCEDURES

Goal: We follow food-purchasing procedures that ensure the meals and snacks served for all children are safe, diverse, and nutritional and contain no harmful chemicals.

❑ Vendors used for food purchasing are licensed and regulated to ensure food safety.

❑ Purchased foods have clear nutritional labeling/information (except whole foods like fresh fruits, vegetables, and bulk grains).

❑ Food-purchasing procedures ensure diversity in flavor, texture, color, and taste.

❑ **Allergies** and modifications (for example, religious preferences or vegetarian diets) are taken into consideration when purchasing food, to ensure all children receive adequate nutrition according to USDA nutritional guidelines.

❑ Purchased fruits and vegetables are fresh, frozen, or packed in water without added sugar or salt.

❑ Foods are purchased in their least processed and packaged forms (for example, fresh fruit rather than fruit snacks).

❑ Prepackaged meals (for example, prepared lasagna or canned stir-fry) are rarely or never used.

❑ More than 50 percent of the grain ingredients and products are whole grain.

❑ Purchased vegetables are primarily dark green and leafy or dark yellow/orange.

❑ Purchased proteins are diverse and include meat, legumes, soy products, and eggs.

Bonus Checklist

❑ Local, fresh produce is purchased whenever possible.

❑ Organic meat, fruits, and vegetables are used when possible.

❑ Organic infant jar or prepared baby food is provided when possible.

❑ Prepared components (for example, canned soup) or foods have five or fewer ingredients.

❑ We discuss our preferences for healthy and nutritious food items with our food vendor(s) each quarter.

❑ The vendor understands our preferences and ensures we receive the healthiest options.

❑ When possible, food is purchased from farmers' markets or local farms.

❑ When possible, food is grown in our program's garden or a community garden.

❑ We evaluate the vitamin and mineral content of food before buying it so children receive many nutrients.

FATS, SUGARS, AND SODIUM

Goal: Through our food purchasing, we ensure that children do not consume many fats, sugars, simple carbohydrates, or sodium.

❑ Purchased food contains very little, if any, saturated or **trans fats**.

❑ Purchased butter or soft margarine *or* products with liquid vegetable oil as a first ingredient have two grams of saturated fat or less, and one gram of trans fat or less per **serving**.

❑ If reduced, low-, or no-fat ingredients or items are purchased, they do not include extra sodium or sugar.

Did you know? Many manufacturers that make reduced, low-, or no-fat ingredients or foods compensate for the missing fat by adding other unhealthy items, like sugar. Look at the food labels on individual products in each brand. Cutting down the amount of fat children consume is good, but they do need some healthy fats in their diet. Reduced-fat products are not always the right choice. Low-carb products should not be bought or served to young children. Not all carbohydrates are bad. **Complex carbohydrates** are very important for optimal growth and development.

❏ Purchased food contains limited sugar, high-fructose corn syrup, or other sugars.

❏ Sugar in any form is not one of the first three ingredients on a food label.

❏ Each unit of purchased food does not contain more than 20 percent of the **daily recommended value** (DRV) (see food label) of sodium.

❏ Purchased meats are at least 90 percent lean, according to the label.

❏ If hot dogs and deli meats are purchased, they are nitrate free.

❏ Only real cheese is purchased (no cheese products).

❏ Purchased cereal does not contain added sugar.

❏ Purchased oatmeal is not instant.

Did you know? Avoid instant oatmeal for two reasons: first, it breaks down faster in the body, turning into sugar quickly. Second, most instant oatmeal includes sugars and food additives. Traditional, slow-cooked oatmeal doesn't take that much longer to cook, and it's cheaper too. On the other hand, instant oatmeal is still a far better choice for breakfast than pastries, doughnuts, or sugared cereals.

Meal and Menu Planning

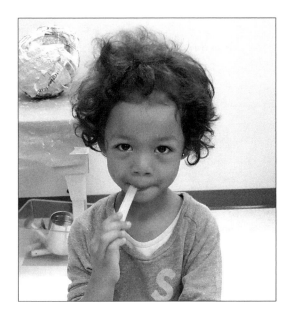

Just because nutritional food is purchased doesn't mean it will still be healthy when it reaches a child's plate. Meal and menu planning, like food preparation (pages 12–15), is important. Without careful planning, meals may provide an imbalance of nutrients. Typical meals and snacks of children in the United States are full of processed or simple carbohydrates, sodium, and sugar and deficient in most vitamins and minerals. Look at the color palate of the foods on a plate—it can sometimes be very telling. If the plate is filled mostly with white or yellow foods, its nutrient value is pretty low. Be aware of the nutritional value (and color) of foods. Plan meals with this in mind so children receive most of the necessary nutrients while they are in care.

Some nutritional choices and practices are harder to change than others. For instance, most people associate celebrations with food. Individual families can make the choice to eat unhealthy foods on occasion (cake to celebrate a birthday, or fast food for dinner on a busy evening). But child care providers should not make these same choices for children while in care. While this may feel uncomfortable or severe, it aligns with the overall goal of most child care programs: to support children's growth, development, and learning in policy and practice at all times. Early care and education programs have the opportunity to increase the health of the children in care and help reverse obesity trends. The childhood obesity epidemic is clear evidence that changes are called for. Early care and education professionals should serve as role models and leaders for families and communities.

MENU-PLANNING PROCEDURES

Goal: We follow menu-planning procedures that ensure children have balanced and nutritious meals and snacks.

❑ Menus are planned to meet USDA MyPlate guidelines for children. (See appendix G in this book to review the guidelines.)

❑ For programs involved in the Children and Adult Care Food Program (CACFP), menus are planned to meet CACFP requirements.

❑ New foods are introduced one at a time on a regular basis.

❑ New foods are offered multiple times (at least seven to ten) before we determine if children will like or eat the item.

Did you know? Introducing new foods can be fun. It doesn't always have to happen at mealtimes. You can plan a fruit-tasting activity or carry out a cooking project. Even better, ask a family member to come and share some cooking with the group. Introducing new foods to young children requires patience. Often it takes ten times or so for children to decide if they like a food or not. Keep at it; don't force it. Helping children develop healthy food preferences is well worth the effort.

❑ Menus for meals and snacks are developed prior to use and shared with families in advance.

❏ Menu substitutions ensure that children are still eating according to the recommended guidelines. Menu substitutions are documented in writing.

❏ Vegetarian or other diet requests are accommodated as long as children receive adequate nutrients.

❏ Meal and snack items are diverse throughout the week and at each meal: different colors, different textures, different tastes, and culturally diverse.

Did you know? Serving culturally diverse foods sometimes requires a little thought. Things like spaghetti and tacos are no longer considered diverse, because they are commonly served in American households and have been Americanized. Serving culturally diverse foods may mean stretching out of your comfort zone. It doesn't have to be complicated. Start with simple things. Offer hummus or tzatziki sauce with vegetables for snack, or prepare fresh salsa as a group. Plan to slowly introduce a variety of flavors to expand children's developing palates.

❏ Children are included in menu planning.

❏ Children are often allowed to make food choices (for example, bananas and peaches are offered, and children are allowed to choose which fruit they prefer).

❏ Desserts are not served.

Did you know? *Gasp!* No dessert, you say? It's true. The idea of saving room for the best part of the meal promotes poor eating habits and unhealthy preferences. It gives all those good foods a bad rap. If you offer a healthy sweet dessert item, like fruit or a low-fat pudding high in calcium, serve it with the meal rather than as a reward for eating the healthy stuff. Remember, you are not saying no desserts ever, but no desserts for children while they are attending your program. The program should focus at all times on healthy child development.

Bonus Checklist

❏ Menus are planned to ensure children receive a variety of **micronutrients** and **macronutrients** each day.

❏ Menus are developed in consultation with a certified/licensed nutritionist or dietitian.

❏ Ingredients and nutritional information for all meals are readily available to family members.

NUTRITIONAL CONTENT OF MEALS AND SNACKS

Goal: The meals and snacks we serve children contain the nutrients they need each day.

❑ A variety of **whole grains/complex carbohydrates** make up at least 50 percent of the carbohydrates served throughout the day.

❑ Proteins served are lean and diverse.

❑ Fruits and vegetables are served without added sugars, cream sauces, or other ingredients that diminish their nutritional value.

❑ Healthy fats, such as nuts (if program allows nuts), olive oil, avocado, and salmon packed in water, are used as ingredients.

❑ Besides milk, foods high in calcium are served daily (for example, cheese, yogurt, spinach, and collard greens).

❑ The milk served has age-appropriate fat content (whole milk for one- to two-year-olds, 1 percent or skim for children age two and older) and is unflavored.

❑ Fruits and vegetables are served at all meals and most snacks.

❑ If juice is served, it is 100 percent fruit and/or vegetable juice and is served no more than once a day (four- to six-ounce **serving** only).

HIGH-SUGAR, HIGH-FAT, AND HIGH-SODIUM FOODS

Goal: Our program rarely, if ever, serves foods high in sugar, fat, or sodium.

❑ Deep-fried foods are not served, including, but not limited to, chicken nuggets, french fries, potato chips, fish sticks, hash browns, or processed french toast sticks.

❑ High-fat or high-sugar foods are not served, including, but not limited to, doughnuts, cakes, sugar-sweetened high-fat yogurt, fruit snacks, candy, or bacon.

❑ Food items with lower nutritional content and high natural sugar, such as corn or potatoes (excluding fried potatoes, which should never be served) are served two or fewer times per week.

❑ Foods served during celebrations also meet these criteria.

FOOD ITEMS FROM OUTSIDE PROGRAM

Goal: All foods served in our program, including foods brought from home or purchased from stores, meet the program's standards.

❑ If families provide meals for children, teachers confirm they are balanced and healthy meals.

❑ If families provide snack items for children, teachers confirm they are nutritious and healthy foods.

❑ Our program keeps nutritious food on hand to supplement children's meals if needed.

❑ Foods brought from home or purchased by families for special events or celebrations meet nutrition and health guidelines (program guidelines).

❑ If children eat meals from an outside vendor regularly or on occasion (for example, on a field trip), those meals are required to meet nutritious and healthy guidelines.

❑ Foods from fast-food restaurants are never allowed in the program for any reason.

Did you know? While some foods from fast-food restaurants may be healthy, fast-food restaurant menus are typically packed with unhealthy, calorie-dense foods. Having an overall **policy** to keep those foods out of your program eliminates the need for you to evaluate each meal brought in from fast-food restaurants. It also minimizes the number of times children are exposed to those restaurants and food choices.

❑ Food requiring refrigeration that is brought from home or outside sources is stored properly (that is, in an actual refrigerator in most cases, even if ice packs are included).

Food Preparation

Food preparation is an important process in a child care program. Being mindful of food safety during food preparation is essential to ensure children's health. And cooking and food preparation are good opportunities to blend ingredients and enhance flavors. Unfortunately, the nutritional value of many foods is lowered or eliminated during cooking. For example, a cooked apple coated with sugars and fats no longer retains its original nutritional value. Preparing foods should not lower their nutritional value. Instead, it should enhance flavor and help children develop a taste for nutritional foods.

FOOD PREPARATION EXPERTISE

Goal: We ensure that those preparing food and meals are trained and knowledgeable about safe and healthful food preparation.

❑ The program has not been cited for any nutritional or food service licensing violations within the past three years. (If violations have occurred, evidence of immediate resolution is required.)

❑ Everyone preparing foods and meals is aware of and trained on:

  ❑ food safety practices including, but not limited to, food handling, correct cooking and storage temperatures, and relevant hygiene practices
  ❑ the nutritional content of the food being prepared and served
  ❑ cooking techniques that contribute to flavor but do not add unwanted sugars, fats, or sodium

FOOD SAFETY

Goal: We consistently follow safe food handling, storage, and preparation practices.

❑ Refrigerators in our program have accurate numerical temperature gauges that are checked for accuracy monthly.

❑ Hot foods are cooled to room temperature before being put in the refrigerator or freezer.

❑ All fruits and vegetables are washed thoroughly before preparation, even if labeled prewashed.

❑ Utensils or surfaces that come in contact with raw meat are washed with soap and hot water immediately after use.

❑ If meat is cooked on site, a meat thermometer is used, and a chart of safe temperatures for cooked meat is posted in a visible location in the kitchen.

❑ Those preparing and cooking food follow strict hand-washing procedures and/or wear gloves to avoid transfer of germs and **cross-contamination**.

Did you know? Cross-contamination can happen easier than you may think. Rinsing raw meat spreads microorganisms on its surface all over your sink. When this happens, everything that sits in your sink becomes contaminated. Applying marinades or juices that touched raw or undercooked meat to fully cooked meat cross-contaminates that cooked meat. Piercing cooked meat with forks or skewers that were used before the meat was fully cooked cross-contaminates the cooked meat.

Failing to wash your hands after handling raw meat is another common cause of cross-contamination. When you touch raw meat and then touch your apron, and then a plate and a spoon that you use to carry already-cooked food, you cross-contaminate your apron, the plate, and the spoon. Using the same cutting boards for raw meats and foods that will be served raw, like some fruits and vegetables, cross-contaminates the foods that will be served raw. Failing to thoroughly wash and dry the exteriors of fruits like watermelons and cantaloupes can introduce contaminants from their surfaces into their flesh when you cut them with a knife.

A little precaution and fastidious practices can save children from potentially harmful germs.

❏ Fruits and vegetables are not used before or after they ripen.

❏ Microwaves are never used for cooking. They can be used for reheating fully cooked foods.

FOOD PREPARATION PRACTICES

Goal: Foods are prepared in ways that retain all or most of their nutritional value and make them appealing and flavorful without added sugars, sodium, and fats.

❏ The recipes we use call for nutritionally sound ingredients. Ingredient substitutions are made when possible to increase the nutritional value of prepared foods.

Did you know? Granted, sometimes ingredient substitutions can alter the flavor or texture of a meal, but that's not always a bad thing. Do a little experimenting—for example, use unsweetened applesauce instead of oil, whole wheat flour instead of white flour, or low-fat plain yogurt instead of sour cream. If experimenting is too costly, many cookbooks provide substitution charts, including the USDA's Menu Magic, which offers tried-and-true substitution tips.

❏ Foods are not fried or are cooked in oils containing **polyunsaturated** or **monounsaturated** fats (refer to labels).

❏ Butter or margarine or butter substitutes are used in limited quantities.

❑ Minimal salt, sugar, or fats are added during cooking or when serving food.

❑ A variety of spices and herbs are used to flavor food and to introduce children to varied flavors.

❑ Fat or grease is removed or drained from meat during cooking.

❑ Skins are washed well and *not* removed from organic fruits and vegetables if they are edible, for example, on apples or potatoes (within food safety guidelines).

❑ Skins from nonorganic fruits and vegetables are removed to limit children's exposures to **pesticides** and other toxins.

❑ Cream-based sauces or condiments are used minimally or not at all.

❑ Skin is removed from all poultry during cooking preparation.

❑ Pans, pots, bowls, and other food preparation supplies are washed between uses to remove oil, fat, or greasy residue and harmful bacteria.

❑ Only low-sodium stock or broth is used in cooking.

Meal and Snack Service

Purchasing and preparing foods that support children's development are important, but all your efforts are useless if children don't eat the food you serve. Make sure food is served in ways that are appetizing and appealing to children without compromising their nutritional value.

MEAL AND SNACK SERVICE

Goal: Meals and snacks of appropriate portion sizes are prepared and served to appeal to children, to make meals enjoyable experiences, and to make it possible for children to serve themselves to the best of their ability (family-style dining).

❑ Children are offered appropriate portions of foods and are assisted in controlling their own portion sizes.

❑ Child-sized dishes and utensils are used so children can manage portions and develop healthy eating habits.

Did you know? Portions and servings are two different things. A portion is how much someone puts on a plate, and it can range greatly, from two cups of macaroni and cheese to three noodles. A serving is how much of an item is recommended by the USDA and Food and Drug Administration (FDA). (Refer to appendix G in this book for the MyPlate serving recommendations for children.) Helping children manage their portions is important. Few people instinctively understand what a serving is, but they can learn to take only what they need—which will often mimic a suggested serving size. A person can always take more if she's still hungry. Doing that is better than piling heaps of food on a plate. To help children, you can model portion control and use serving utensils that encourage taking appropriate portions. In a culture of oversized portions, where "More is better" seems to be our mantra, portion control is an important lifelong skill.

❑ Enough food is provided so all children and teachers can have adequate servings of everything.

❑ Children are encouraged to serve themselves so they can begin to regulate and choose their own portions.

❑ The food looks appetizing.

Did you know? Adults don't like to eat food that doesn't look appetizing—children are no different. Take a few simple steps to make sure food is appealing: serve foods at safe temperatures, cook green vegetables in a way that retains their vibrant color, and provide a variety of colorful healthy foods at each meal.

❑ Salt, sugar, and fats are not separately available to add after food has been prepared.

Section 2

Healthy Eating Habits for Infants

The nutrition infants receive contributes significantly to their overall healthy physical and mental development. The **nutrients** growing fetuses receive in the womb affect children's long-term growth, including their brain cells and cognitive development. Many national organizations and research studies support these points. For instance, according to the federal Centers for Disease Control and Prevention (CDC) (2010), babies and mothers experience many benefits from breast-feeding. Breast milk is easy to digest and contains antibodies that can protect infants from bacterial and viral infections. Research also indicates that women who breast-feed may have lower rates of certain breast and ovarian cancers. Additional research cited in National Scientific Council on the Developing Child and National Forum on Early Childhood Policy and Programs report "The Foundations of Lifelong Health Are Built in Early Childhood" (2010) states:

> Health at every stage of the life course is influenced by nutrition, beginning with the mother's pre-conception nutritional status, extending through pregnancy to early infant feeding and weaning, and continuing with diet and activity throughout childhood and into adult life.
>
> Inadequate maternal nutrition during pregnancy is associated with a range of undesirable outcomes in the offspring, including obesity in childhood and adulthood as well as subsequent hypertension and cardiovascular disease. (10–11)

How infants are fed contributes to healthy eating habits. For example, if they do not have regular and predictable meals, they may develop snacking tendencies or be tempted to hoard food. If they are overfed, they may learn to ignore internal cues that they are full. Infants who are fed solids too early may develop **allergies** or have difficulty eating if their reflexes aren't fully developed (these reflexes develop between four and six months). Studies also indicate that children who are breast-fed have a 22 percent lower chance of becoming obese than children who are not breast-fed (White House Task Force on Childhood Obesity 2010). Amazingly, often these effects don't show up until adolescence, demonstrating once again that much of the impact of early childhood occurs long after a child grows up.

Of course, child care providers cannot make nutrition decisions for pregnant mothers. You certainly should not demand specific nutritional choices or tell new mothers to breast-feed. It is important that teachers provide factual information and resources to families and use policies and practices that actively support them when they make nutritional choices for their infants.

This section will address:

- Breast-feeding: Breast or bottle feeding is the first nutritional decision families make after a child is born. Understanding the value of breast-feeding and having resources and practices to support mothers who choose to is an important part of establishing early positive nutrition patterns.

- Infant nutrition practices: Habits and preferences begin in infancy; establishing healthy practices from the start can make a lasting impact.

- Infant meals: Infants are dependent on the adults around them to expose them to nutritious and healthy foods.

Breast-Feeding

The benefits of breast-feeding versus formula feeding have been discussed for decades. As scientific knowledge has evolved, our society's feelings about breast-feeding have changed. Women's roles have also changed significantly in the past century. These factors work together to influence women's choices about breast-feeding. The evidence is conclusive that breast-feeding offers significant advantages over formula feeding. But women do not breast-feed for many reasons. For instance, some women are unsure how to do so successfully or feel self-conscious about breast-feeding in public. Many women's work schedules do not allow them to express breast milk at work (although a recent amendment to the Fair Labor Standards Act (FLSA) requires employers to provide reasonable break time and private space to express breast milk). Some women cannot breast-feed for medical reasons.

Fortunately, child care programs can lessen some of the challenges women face in feeding their infants. Put aside your personal feelings about breast-feeding. Instead, offer support and information to families. Formula feeding is not harmful to children, and some mothers simply can't breast feed, so it's important not to judge mothers who do not breast-feed. Making sure families have correct information before they make their choice is an important part your child care program can play.

BREAST-FEEDING

Goal: We support breast-feeding in our program.

❑ The program offers new or pregnant mothers reliable information about the benefits of breast-feeding.

❑ The program has a private and comfortable space set aside for mothers to use for breast-feeding or expressing breast milk on-site.

Did you know? Often, a space for breast-feeding mothers is an afterthought. Sometimes a chair is put in the nap area, or the women's restroom is used and a sign put on the door while a mother uses it. Not all programs have the luxury of setting aside a space for the sole purpose of breast-feeding. But it's important to give some thought and attention to providing a regular space. It should be calming and welcoming and include information about where to rent or buy a breast pump, a storage area for breast pumps, an outlet, and a sink for hand washing. Giving some attention to this space underscores your program's respect and support for breast-feeding mothers.

❑ Equipment (for example, a refrigerator and freezer with required and reliable temperatures, safe warming devices, and labels) is readily available to store and prepare bottles of freshly expressed and frozen breast milk. (See appendix J in this book to review breast milk handling and storage recommendations.)

❑ If a child is breast-fed during the day, backup bottles of expressed milk are stored in case the mother is delayed for a feeding.

❑ Families are not judged on their decision or ability to breast-feed or formula feed their infants.

Bonus Checklist

❑ The program organizes and/or supports breast-feeding mentors or support groups.

Infant Nutrition Practices

The nutrition infants receive affects their ability to thrive and grow to their fullest potential. Child care programs need intentional practices and procedures that contribute to infants' nutrition and support development of partnerships between families and teachers. Everyone must contribute to open communication about children's nutrition. Establishing practices and procedures helps your program maintain consistent, quality approaches to nutrition.

INFANT NUTRITION PRACTICES

Goal: We follow infant nutritional practices that meet nutritional goals for infants, and we develop partnerships between teachers and families regarding nutrition.

❑ A nutritional plan is on file for each infant (some states require a nutritional plan; if yours does not, see appendix I in this book for a reproducible sample).

❑ Every day, the type and amount of food each infant consumes is recorded and shared with the infant's family.

❑ Teachers feed infants based on their individual needs and routines.

> **Did you know?** Some families request that their infants be put on feeding schedules. You can try to accommodate this request if you choose. However, breast milk/formula or food should never be withheld from an obviously hungry infant. An infant's cues should never be ignored. Ignoring their cries of hunger establishes unhealthy patterns and sends mixed messages to them. If families know how your program handles this situation up front, they will form a partnership with you more easily.

❑ Food safety and storage procedures are strictly followed for all infant foods and fluids.

❑ Families' cultural preferences and practices are always considered and respected when making decisions about infant foods.

Infant Meals

Although infants cannot verbalize their preferences or make choices about their nutrition, their preferences and choices are being formed from their very first days. These can shape their lifelong habits. For example, infants who are regularly overfed often continue to overeat throughout their lifetime; they are less able to sense their own bodies' cues. Infants who are fed sweet fruits or desserts as their first foods may develop preferences for sweet above other flavors. Infants grow and develop rapidly, and their bodies need a range of nutrients to thrive. Infants' first year of development is critical; there's no time for substituting **nutritionally void** foods for **nutritious** foods.

INFANT FLUIDS AND BOTTLES

Goal: All liquids served to infants are nutritious, meet developmental needs, and serve as a foundation for lifelong healthy eating habits.

❑ Only milk or formula is served in bottles (no juice).

❑ Formula served to infants is iron fortified (unless a doctor recommends otherwise in writing).

❑ Formula or milk is never diluted.

❑ Teachers are trained on proper storage (freezer or refrigeration) and handling of breast milk and formula by an expert source. (See appendix J in this book to review breast milk handling and storage recommendations.)

❑ A system has been established for differentiating breast milk bottles from formula bottles.

❑ All bottles are labeled with the infant's name.

❑ Whenever infants drink from bottles, they are always held by a teacher.

Did you know? Bottle safety is mandatory. Bottles must never be propped up. Bottles must never be given to children in swings, cribs, or other devices. Children are never allowed to walk around with bottles.

❑ Bottles are used only to relieve hunger (that is, they should not be provided because infants are fussy and teachers cannot attend to them).

❑ Water is given only to infants six months or older.

INFANT FOOD

Goal: Foods served to infants are nutritious and support the early development of healthy eating habits.

❑ Food, including infant cereal, is not introduced any earlier than four months unless a physician's request is provided in writing (six months is ideal for breast-fed infants).

❑ Teachers know what indicators or cues to look for that signal infants are ready to try solid food.

❑ When infants begin eating solids, one new food is introduced at a time (this should be part of the nutritional plan and determined in partnership with families).

❑ Infant cereal served is iron fortified (unless a doctor recommends otherwise in writing).

❑ If jarred food is to be served, it is never served directly out of the jar unless the whole jar will be used. Used utensils never come in contact with the food in the jar. The remaining food is stored according to directions on the label.

❑ If families provide food, the program offers information on appropriate nutrition for infants.

❑ Infants have consistent teachers so the infants' hunger cues can be recognized.

❑ Infants are never given sweet desserts from jars or as table food.

❑ Table foods are introduced one at a time over three to five days. This allows time to notice any allergic reactions.

❑ Infants' emerging self-feeding skills are nurtured and supported when table foods are introduced.

Did you know? Being able to feed oneself is an important milestone in a child's life. You can support this emerging skill by offering easy-to-grasp foods in bite-sized pieces. Use large, easy-to-grip utensils. Let the child have access to food (yes, it will be dumped or spilled a few times). Once infants can feed themselves, they can also regulate their portions and respond to their own bodily cues.

Bonus Checklist

❑ The program prepares nutritious infant food on-site.

Section 3

Healthy Eating Habits for Children

Early childhood environments are optimal places to start children's knowledge of food. According to the American Academy of Pediatrics (2010), American Public Health Association, and National Resource Center for Health and Safety in Child Care and Early Education, "Children can learn healthy eating habits and be better equipped to maintain a healthy weight if they eat nourishing food while attending early care and education settings and if they are allowed to feed themselves and determine the amount of food they ingest at any one sitting" (13).

Genetics influence a child's growth and development, and so do early experiences: "As children begin to eat at the family table and with other children in child care settings, they become familiar with an ever-widening variety of tastes and textures. Through this process, they form strong and lasting opinions about what foods and beverages are proper and preferred for meals, snacks, and celebrations" (Nitzke et al. 2010, 2).

This section will address:

- Beverages: Beverages are often overlooked when considering nutrition, but they are often calorie dense and lack any nutrients.
- Mealtime behaviors: Developing mealtime behaviors that support healthy eating habits is as important as having access to nutritious food.

Beverages

Whenever nutrition is discussed, the focus is primarily on food. However, beverages contribute a lot to a person's daily caloric, sugar, sodium, and vitamin intake as well. Fruit juice with added sugar, sodas, and energy drinks add significant calories and food additives to a daily diet. Some of these drinks can even be nutritionally harmful. It is important that children (and adults) consume healthy beverages so they get the nutrients they need, without added calories, and develop preferences for them.

Most important, water is an essential component of child and adult diets. Our culture has so many beverage choices that drinking plain water has become less common. Bottled water has become more popular than tap water. Unfortunately, this is not good for the environment or children's health. Most bottled water is missing some of the nutritional benefits of tap water, for example, fluoride. Child care programs should nurture children's taste for safe tap water.

BEVERAGES

Goal: All fluids consumed by children meet their nutritional needs and do not contain empty calories or harmful additives.

❑ After children are weaned from bottles, they are given unflavored whole milk until they are twenty-four months old. (Soy, rice, or other milk substitutes without added sugars are acceptable for children with documented **allergies** or family cultural preferences.)

❑ Children over twenty-four months of age are given low or nonfat, unflavored milk. (Soy, rice, or other milk substitutes without added sugars are acceptable for children with documented allergies or family cultural preferences.)

❑ Children do not drink more than thirty-two ounces of cow's milk a day (although child care programs cannot fully regulate this, they can ensure children do not drink more than this amount in their program).

❑ Unflavored and fluoridated water is available and accessible at all times to children over age twelve months (exceptions are made if the city does not have fluoridated water and children receive fluoride in other ways).

❑ Juice is served no more than once a day (four- to six-ounce **serving**).

❑ All juices served are 100 percent fruit juice and contain no added sugars or artificial sweeteners.

❑ Children in toddler, preschool, or school-age programs are never given bottles. (Exception can be made for children transitioning to toddler programs if a plan is in place to eventually eliminate the use of the bottle. The child must sit with a teacher while drinking from the bottle.)

❑ For toddlers only: If sippy cups are used, they are used only during mealtime. Children must be seated to use them. The sippy cups are used only as a transition from bottles to cups and only in toddler programs.

❑ Bottled water is used only when untested or harmful water is the only other choice.

Mealtime Behaviors

How people eat is often as important as what they eat. In the past, meals took time to prepare, and families gathered around a table to eat them together. As they ate their food, they spent time talking. Often this was a bonding experience. It also helped people stay healthy. By eating food they had prepared themselves, they knew what ingredients went into it. Eating together encouraged eating slowly, which aided digestion and helped them know if they were full or still hungry. Today the average family's schedules and the convenience of restaurant meals have decreased the time people spend preparing and eating food. Further, restaurant foods are often high in additives (most notably sodium), sugars, and fats. These ingredients can affect immediate and long-term health and often lead to overeating and weight gain.

Teachers can help children read their own bodies' cues so they know how full or hungry they are. To that end, children should be offered food at regular intervals throughout the day. Additionally, children should not be required to eat when they aren't hungry. They should not develop a habit of snacking throughout the day, either. Food should be used to give their bodies energy. It should not be treated as a reward or a **punishment**. Children need food for energy, and most of them eagerly choose to eat at allotted times. If a child is not eating meals, you should discuss this immediately with the child's family. Consistent teacher-child relationships enable you to recognize and understand children's eating patterns as they change and develop in the early years.

MEALTIME BEHAVIORS

Goal: When children have meals and snacks while in the program, they learn healthy eating habits and mealtime behaviors that contribute to their health and wellness.

- ❑ If adults are helping children serve themselves, **portion** sizes provided are child appropriate.

- ❑ Meals and snacks are served **family style**.

- ❑ Meal and snack times are pleasant social experiences.

- ❑ Children are never required to clean their plates. They are encouraged to eat only until they are full.

- ❑ Children have consistent teachers who know each child's eating habits and preferences and can recognize each child's body cues.

- ❑ A minimum of twenty minutes is allotted for snacktime. This does not include hand washing or food service.

- ❑ A minimum of thirty minutes is allotted for each meal. This does not include hand washing or food service.

Did you know? Part of developing healthy eating habits is learning to enjoy meals and snacktime. If they are always rushed, then children won't learn to appreciate the experience. In addition, digestion takes time. Overeating often occurs when meals are rushed. Giving your body enough time to send the message to your brain that you are full is an important habit to develop.

❑ Children are never forced to eat.

❑ Food, nutrition, and healthy eating habits are discussed during meals and snacktime.

❑ Unless it is part of a curriculum activity, children and adults consume food only during meals or snacktime.

❑ Children and adults consume food only while seated at a table.

❑ Children are encouraged to eat a variety of foods at each meal rather than a single food item.

❑ Children are allowed to leave the table when they are finished eating.

Section 4

Program Approach to Nutrition

You can help children develop positive, healthy attitudes toward food and eating that can last a lifetime. What you choose to focus on and teach, as well as what you don't teach, influences children's development now and in the future. You also teach through modeling and your own actions. Model healthy behaviors. Do not minimize the impact your own behaviors have on the children in your care.

Eating fast food in front of children, making a face when vegetables are served, even using soda pop or candy containers as props in dramatic play areas influence how children feel about food. Teachers who require children to clean their plates or who use food as a **punishment** or reward are using food in inappropriate ways. These actions can foster unhealthy feelings and attitudes toward food. Food's sole purpose is to nourish and provide energy.

According to Jeanette Betancourt, Sesame Workshop's vice president of Outreach and Educational Practices, "By the time a child is between two and four years old, her eating habits are largely shaped. If she reaches the age of five without learning about healthy eating, the chances of her developing poor nutritional habits and attitudes are significantly increased" (as quoted in Greenbush Healthy Living 2012).

This section will address:

- Modeling and teaching: Children will do as you do. Knowing how to model and teach healthy eating habits and nutrition throughout the day can make a big impression on young learners.

- Nutrition education: Nutrition education is much more than teaching about the food groups. There are bountiful ideas and resources to enrich your daily lesson plan.

Modeling and Teaching

Children learn from what they see and experience. If you model and teach healthy eating habits and nutrition, then these lessons have a significant impact on children's lifelong approach to food and nutrition. We know that having books in a classroom, reading stories out loud, engaging children in conversation, and singing songs and rhymes contribute to children's language development even before they can speak. Similarly, consistent and positive approaches to teaching nutrition throughout the day contribute to children's physical development and their relationships to food.

TEACHER MODELING BEHAVIORS

Goal: We model positive and healthy eating habits and nutrition.

❑ Teachers and children sit at the table together to eat meals and snacks.

❑ Teachers' comments and body language about food are positive and focus on good nutrition.

❑ Teachers model self-feeding and healthy eating behaviors, such as chewing slowly, not adding salt or sugar, and eating a variety of healthy foods.

❑ Teachers model a positive approach to trying new foods.

❑ Teachers do not perpetuate food myths, such as "carbs make you fat" or "vegetables are rabbit food."

❑ Teachers do not describe people using weight-related terms like *fat*, *chubby*, *thin*, or *skinny*.

❑ Teachers help children express dislike of a food positively (for example, "I don't like it yet") rather than in ways that may influence other children's willingness to try a food.

❑ Teachers are held to the same nutritional standards as children and families. If this is not possible or practical, then:

> ❑ Teachers do not eat unhealthy food in front of children, for example, soda pop, chips, candy, or fast food.
> ❑ If teachers bring their own food to eat, they eat away from the children.
> ❑ If the center has vending machines, they are not visible to the children.
> ❑ A private space is available for teachers to eat away from children if they choose.

TEACHING HEALTHY EATING HABITS

Goal: Children in our program learn about nutrition and healthful eating throughout the day in a variety of ways.

❑ Teachers engage in positive conversations about nutrition and health during meals and snacktime and spontaneously during other parts of the day.

❑ Food is never withheld from children for behavior-related reasons. This includes specialty items served at special events or celebrations.

❑ Children are encouraged, but not required, to try new foods.

❑ Children are not required to clean their plates.

❑ Teachers never use food or beverages as punishment or reward.

Did you know? Think about it. If you tell children they'll get a piece of candy if they clean up, what do they learn from that? Yes, you will probably get them to clean up, but you will also teach them that they should only clean for a reward and that candy is something to work for. Conversely, if you punish them by forcing them to eat all of their lima beans, you may create a long-term aversion to a healthy and **nutritious** food. Many other ways exist to guide children's behavior; leave food out of it.

❑ Teachers help children identify what *full* and *hungry* mean and use these terms in meaningful ways during mealtime.

❑ Teachers discuss the differences between thirst and hunger. (Many young children confuse thirst with hunger and eat when a glass of water would actually meet their needs.)

Nutrition Education

Education about nutrition and eating is rarely intentional and frequently occurs only at meals or snacktimes. For these lessons to fully influence children's development and life choices, they must be taught throughout the day. As you know, physical development is one of the primary developmental domains. To address it, child care programs typically focus on large- and small-motor development. But nutrition and healthy eating habits are important parts of physical development. Weave developmentally appropriate nutrition education into children's daily experience. Doing so can make a positive impact on their overall physical development.

THE LEARNING ENVIRONMENT

Goal: Our learning environment reflects an intentional focus on nutrition and healthy eating.

❑ Nutrition is part of the daily learning environment rather than a special focus that comes and goes.

❑ Positive examples of good nutrition and healthy eating habits are evident in the learning environment.

❑ Visible examples of positive nutrition and healthy eating habits can be found in many learning areas.

> **Did you know?** You can focus on nutrition in the learning environment in many ways: posters or collages showing children and families enjoying healthy foods, child-planted gardens, healthy food props and menus, class-written stories about healthy food, and children's books about nutrition.

❑ There are no unhealthy models in the classroom, such as pictures of fast-food restaurant signs, or soda pop containers and doughnut boxes in dramatic play.

❑ The learning environment shows evidence of prior learning and ongoing focus on nutrition.

❑ Children are never intentionally exposed to advertisements for unhealthy food during the program.

❑ Dramatic play themes and props offer daily opportunities to learn and explore healthy eating habits and nutrition.

NUTRITION CURRICULUM

Goal: Teachers intentionally plan activities that teach good nutrition and healthy eating. Daily lesson plans, curriculum, and/or children's activities reflect this.

❑ Education on nutrition and healthy eating habits is part of each weekly lesson plan for all ages.

❑ We provide daily opportunities for children to learn about making good choices and decisions.

> **Did you know?** While decision-making skills influence children's nutrition, they do not have to be taught only during meals and snacktime. You can promote decision making throughout the day whether it's during a peer interaction or a group activity. Allowing children to make decisions for themselves and their bodies is important. It contributes to good nutrition as well as good self-care.

❑ The program has a food garden. The children help care for it weekly in the growing season.

❑ Healthy cooking or food-related projects are part of the weekly plan. Children can explore topics like the origins of food, the taste of foods prepared differently, and the food groups.

❑ We occasionally have guests and field trips to places related to healthy eating and nutrition. These may include a local chef or restaurant, a farmer/gardener or farm/garden, a grocery store or farmers' market, even the program's kitchen, if children don't regularly use it.

❑ Our nutrition learning includes but is not necessarily limited to:
   ❑ the value of good nutrition
   ❑ the different food groups
   ❑ understanding the body's energy needs and making nutrition choices accordingly
   ❑ where foods are from and how they are prepared

Bonus Checklist

❑ We use a research-based nutrition curriculum to guide our educational activities. A physical development curriculum that addresses nutrition and healthy eating is also acceptable.

Section 5

Nutrition Education and Resources for Families

When children and families do not make healthy food choices, it is often because they are misinformed or overwhelmed by the various sources of information. If a family lacks the best information, how can they make the right choices for their children? Fortunately, because of recent national focus on nutrition, many credible resources are now available to educate and guide adults. Great resources also exist for children. You can ensure that families have continuous access to reliable information and resources.

This section will address:

- Family resources and support: Providing resources and identifying community support for families related to healthy eating habits and nutrition helps strengthen the partnership between families and the program and can positively influence families' nutrition practices at home.

- Program resources: Teachers always appreciate reliable and useful resources. Making resources available to teachers related to healthy eating habits and nutrition increases the likelihood that they can effectively teach and instill healthy habits.

Family Resources and Support

Child care programs cannot choose how or what to feed pregnant mothers or how families nourish their children at home. But they do have a role to play in families' food choices: families often look to providers for information about child development. While only medical and nutrition professionals have expertise on prenatal, infant, and child nutrition, you can inform and influence families nonetheless. Information from accurate and trusted resources is most likely to be well received. It may help families make changes to support their developing children.

SUPPORTING FAMILIES

Goal: Our program provides families with access to credible and relevant resources and information on nutrition and healthy eating to help them make informed decisions about health and nutrition.

❏ Information is provided to families about the program's nutritional policies and practices when they enroll.

❏ Ongoing education and information on nutrition is provided to families.

❏ Our program newsletter includes a regular section on nutrition and healthy eating.

❏ Our teachers work to develop a partnership with families on children's healthy eating habits and nutrition.

❏ Our program invites families to be involved in, lead, or learn about our nutrition curriculum.

❏ At least one of our community resource partners focuses on educating or supporting families about infant and/or pregnancy nutrition.

❏ The program is in contact with the local Women, Infant, and Children (WIC) office and provides information about WIC to all families.

❏ If food is served at family events, then our program serves or encourages healthy foods and drinks.

Bonus Checklist

❏ Our program partners with community resources to promote nutrition and healthy eating habits.

❏ The program does not host or sponsor fundraisers that promote non-nutritious food.

PRENATAL AND INFANT NUTRITION SUPPORT AND RESOURCES

Goal: Our program offers information and resources for families so they can make informed decisions about nutrition during pregnancy and infancy.

❑ When pregnant families enroll in the program, they are offered information about nutrition during pregnancy and during the time a mother is breast-feeding.

❑ When pregnant families enroll in the program, they are offered information about the program's infant feeding policies, including breast-feeding support.

❑ The program makes resources on prenatal nutrition available. Family members know how to access these resources.

Bonus Checklist

❑ A lactation consultant is available to family members.

❑ A registered dietitian is available to families to answer child nutrition questions about picky eating, childhood obesity, healthful snack choices, and other topics.

Program Resources

Child care programs and providers should be trusted and reliable resources on child development for families. Families often look to their provider first for such information. Of course, it's unlikely you'll know every fact about every topic. If you have access to current, reliable, and relevant resources, the families you serve can learn what they need to know, when they need to know it.

PROGRAM RESOURCES

Goal: Our program has reliable and relevant resources about nutrition and healthy eating for families and teachers to use.

❑ Books, DVDs, and/or other nutrition resources are available in our family lending library.

❑ Books, DVDs, and/or other nutrition resources are available in our teacher resource library.

❑ We have developed a relationship with a licensed child dietitian. We consult with the dietitian as needed.

❑ The program provides resources so teachers can effectively incorporate nutrition into their lesson plans.

Bonus Checklist

❑ A licensed dietitian is available to the program to help develop menus, train teachers, and provide training.

❑ The program hosts nutrition-related events, such as community health fairs or healthy-cooking classes.

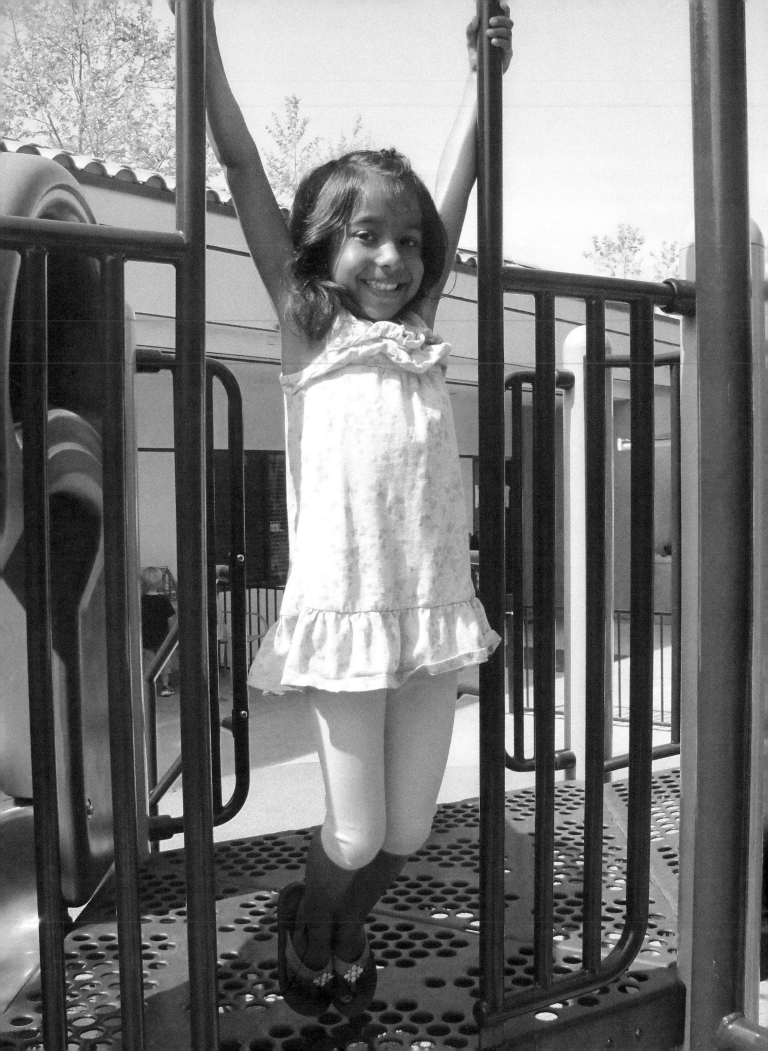

Part 2

Physical Activity and Fitness

When adults reminisce about their childhood, they often recall memories of **physical activities**:

"We used to ride our bikes from sunup to sundown."

"We'd all just meet at the vacant lot and play baseball for hours every weekend."

"We walked over five miles to school, uphill both ways."

While that last one is a famous exaggeration, such memories remind you of what most teachers think of as a right of childhood: free, unscheduled playtime. Today children experience less of this type of play and less physical activity overall. The causes are many: children's extracurricular schedules, access to electronic media, neighborhood safety, organized competitive sports for young children, and less in-school physical education and/or recess. When today's children become adults, what will they remember when they reflect on their childhoods? Will they remember active play experiences, or will they recall only video games, MP3 players, and smartphones?

The Obesity Epidemic

National attention on childhood obesity has increased significantly in the past few years. The statistics on obesity in general and on childhood obesity specifically are shocking. According to the Centers for Disease Control and Prevention (CDC), childhood obesity has more than tripled in the past thirty years. Obesity among children six to eleven years old increased from 6.5 percent in 1980 to 19.6 percent in 2008. Obesity among adolescents twelve to nineteen years old increased from 5.0 percent to 18.1 percent (Ogden and Carroll 2010). And these figures are only for people categorized as obese. Millions of children are not obese but are still considered overweight.

Equally disturbing, as a nation we spend $150 billion every year to treat obesity-related conditions directly and indirectly. That cost is growing (Shaping America's Youth 2012). First Lady Michelle Obama has focused on obesity with her Let's Move! campaign. Its ambitious goal is to end childhood obesity within a generation. She is motivated by disheartening research-based observations like the following, stated by former surgeon general Richard Carmana: "For the first time in American history, our children's life expectancy may be shorter than their parents" (AHA 2011).

Obesity contributes to many problems, including physical limitations, illness, and emotional challenges. More and more professional communities are examining how this epidemic is affecting them and what they can do about it. Even the U.S. military has raised concerns about the current health of America's youth. A report generated by Mission: Readiness (2009), a nonprofit national security organization, states that 75 percent of young people in the United States are ineligible to serve their country. They have either failed to graduate from high school, engaged in criminal activity, or are physically or mentally unfit.

SCREEN TIME AND MEDIA USE

A focus on screen time is an important component of any physical activity initiative for young children. Screen time is any time spent in front of an electronic screen, including televisions and computers. **Passive media** refers to time spent watching screens that does not require interaction, including most television shows and movies. **Interactive media** refers to time in front of screens that requires the viewer to interact, for example, computer games, gaming consoles, or e-readers.

According to the Kaiser Family Foundation (KFF),

- two-thirds of infants and toddlers watch a screen an average of two hours a day;

- children under the age of six watch an average of about two hours of screen media a day, primarily television and videos or DVDs;

- children and teens age eight to eighteen spend nearly four hours a day in front of a television screen and almost two more hours on the computer (outside of doing schoolwork) and playing video games. (2004)

The recently released policy statement of the American Academy of Pediatrics (AAP) (2011) on media use by children under age two states that 90 percent of parents report their children watch some form of electronic media (1040). Media choices are rapidly increasing. With almost nonstop access, children are more exposed to screens than ever before. While not all screen time is bad, too much screen time, exposure to poor-quality, passive media, and any screen time before age two can adversely affect growing children. The AAP's statement says, "Media use has been associated with obesity, sleep issues, aggressive behaviors, and attention issues in preschool- and school-aged children" (1043). Screen time also limits children's opportunities for adult-child or peer interactions. Most relevant to this book, sitting in front of a screen for prolonged periods of time contributes to a **sedentary** lifestyle and limits physical activity. Because exposure to screens clearly negatively affects children's health, the AAP's revised policy statement strongly recommends no screen time for children under age two. This includes a television playing in the background.

Note: A significant amount of research on screen time, electronic technology, and media use in young children is available. This book addresses screen time only in relation to physical activity and **fitness**.

Solutions

Fortunately, these trends can be turned around. Along with increased attention to nutrition and healthy eating, a comprehensive and purposeful approach toward physical activity and fitness is needed. The key finding of the first surgeon general's report on physical activity (*Physical Activity and Health: A Report of the Surgeon General Executive Summary*) is that all individuals can benefit from moderate increases in physical activity (US HHS, CDC, and PCPFS 1996). For many years people believed a "no pain, no gain" approach to **exercise** was the only way they could benefit from physical activity. The surgeon general's report dispels this myth. **Moderate activity**, such as walking for thirty minutes four or five days a week (for adults), or participating in physical play an hour a day (for young children)—all at once *or* in intervals—can significantly improve physical and mental health and overall fitness. (See appendix F in this book to review examples of moderate activities for young children.) This news makes having a healthy, active lifestyle a realistic and achievable goal.

MORE THAN JUST PHYSICAL HEALTH

It is worthwhile to mention that physical activity can have a significant impact beyond physical health. Much research has been done on the positive impact of exercise on mental health. Convinced by current research, many physicians now prescribe exercise as part of their treatment plans for anxiety, depression, and even addiction. Moderate physical activity is associated with long life, less injury, longer mobility, and lower rates of cardiovascular and other debilitating diseases (CDC 1997). Physical activity is also positively correlated with learning. Children who can **exercise** throughout their day often show increased cognitive skills and academic performance, and "studies continue to show that children who are physically active in their early years have a significantly greater chance of achieving success in school" (MLRC 2004). Physical activity can contribute to brain alertness, learning readiness, attention, and engagement.

WHAT SHOULD THE EARLY CARE AND EDUCATION COMMUNITY DO?

National attention is helpful, and reports on exercise and its positive effects are compelling. But they won't make a difference unless you put the research findings and recommendations into practice every day. Child care programs are in a unique position to support physical activity and exercise habits. Unfortunately, many programs are not doing so. According to many reports, children in child care spend an average of 70 to 87 percent of their time in sedentary activities (AAP, APHA, and NRC 2010). This is an easily reversible situation and one the early childhood community should be dedicated to improving. Large-motor play is an important aspect of child care programs. It should not be reduced to make room for more content study or increased academic focus. Playtime should not be *just* about running around freely (although this is important). It's an opportunity to build important physical skills such as coordination, balance, flexibility, endurance, and strength, and behavioral skills like goal setting, self-assessment, and physical confidence. **Structured** and **unstructured activities** are both important. Ensure that children have ample physical activity opportunities throughout each day in engaging and interesting environments, both indoors and outside. Provide resources and support to families. Nurture a love of physical activity. When you do so, you support the development of lifelong habits of physical activity.

Physical activity needn't occur in isolation. Like development in all learning domains, physical development happens alongside social and emotional, cognitive, literacy, and other development domains. Physical activity can focus on several aspects of physical development at the same time. For instance, an active game of Simon Says can build coordination, muscle control, and ability to follow directions. A relay race that requires passing a baton can develop hand-eye coordination, endurance, and peer relationships. Time spent on their tummies can increase infants' strength and coordination.

You should be aware of the harmful images and stereotypes of bodies that children may see or hear. From a young age, they should learn healthy attitudes about body image. They should not be exposed to advertising or unrealistic images. Their environments should be free from teasing, labeling, and other behaviors that diminish confidence. Children should enjoy physical activity without worrying about meeting certain standards and images or participating in constant competition.

Of course, you have your own attitudes and habits toward physical activity. But when working with and modeling for children, all adults should engage in as much activity as they safely can. You don't try to teach literacy without reading to children and demonstrating your own love for reading. So why teach physical development differently? You should model best practices for physical activity, teaching children not just by telling but also by doing.

Section 6

Developing Physical Activity and Fitness Habits in Children

Most early childhood programs identify four or more primary domains of development: cognitive, social, emotional, and physical. Physical development is often unconsciously relegated to the bottom of the priority list when teachers plan curriculum and learning activities. Outdoor free play is often the only time scheduled for physical development. More often than not, the activities children engage in during this time are **unstructured**. Granted, unstructured outdoor playtime is important, but it is equally important to offer **planned** physical development opportunities daily. This allows you to nurture

- physical development skills, such as endurance, agility, and flexibility,

- healthy bodies, including muscle strength, bone strength, and cardiovascular health, and

- behavioral skills related to physical development, like goal setting and **internal motivation**.

Children must engage in **physical activity** from infancy to fully develop their muscles, bones, and motor skills. Physical activity produces many health benefits, such as improved sleep patterns, increase in positive moods, minimized risk of disease, and improved cardiovascular **fitness**. Furthermore, physical activity can have a positive impact on cognitive development and learning.

Unfortunately, the behaviors of many children do not meet the moderate standards of the surgeon general or the basic recommendations of the National Association for Sport and Physical Education (NASPE). (These standards help minimize health risks, increase physical abilities, improve mental health, and contribute to learning. See appendix B in this book to review NASPE's recommendations.) According to the surgeon general's (1999) report *Physical Activity and Health*, 60 percent of people in the United States are not regularly active, and 25 percent are not active at all.

As an early childhood educator, you know that many lifelong behaviors and habits begin in early childhood. Even moderate physical activity can improve a person's overall health. (See appendix F in this book for examples of moderate and vigorous activities for young children.) You can help build a healthy foundation for each child's life by planning appropriate daily physical activity and supporting the development of physical activity habits.

This section will address:

- Promoting physical activity and fitness: It is important to expose children to a variety of structured and unstructured physical activity and fitness to develop multiple skills, muscles, and abilities. This requires programs to plan less time doing sedentary activities, including television and computers, and spending more time in spaces that can accommodate movement.

Promoting Physical Activity and Fitness

Physical activity and **fitness** should be promoted throughout the day. Children should have many opportunities, both **structured** and **unstructured**, to engage in experiences that promote their physical development. Participation should be encouraged, activities should be collaborative rather than competitive, and activities should spark the diverse interests of children. Child care programs should encourage children to spend much of their time on active and interactive activities. You and your program should value and prioritize physical activity and fitness as an integral part of your overall curriculum.

THE DAILY SCHEDULE

Goal: Children have daily opportunities for physical activity and fitness in our program.

❑ Children's physical development is a daily focus.

❑ Daily schedules include at least two physical activity experiences. At least one should be outside, weather permitting. (Half-day programs need at least one experience.)

❑ Indoor physical activities and resources are planned in case of bad weather.

❑ Some of the time scheduled for physical activity includes structured activities.

❑ Some of the time scheduled for physical activity includes time for free choice and movement.

SCREEN TIME AND MEDIA USE

Goal: Screen time is limited and developmentally appropriate.

❑ The program does not use television or movies during the day, even in bad weather.

❑ Computer stations or centers are available only to children over age two (if at all) and no more than thirty minutes per day.

❑ Video games are not part of the daily schedule or learning environment.

❑ No child under age two is exposed to any type of media screen.

❑ Interactive technology (for example, stories on tape, recording devices, tablets, e-readers) is used only to support learning.

Did you know? If electronic technology is used in an early care and education environment, it should be used purposefully and meaningfully, integrated into the children's day rather than used for isolated activities. For example, children building a city in the block area can look up maps or building resources on a tablet computer. Children planting a garden can watch an on-screen demonstration of the life cycle of a seed. Children interested in reading can listen to stories on CD. This approach to technology promotes it as a tool rather than as entertainment. It also encourages children to interact while using technology.

❑ Teachers do not have the television on in the background of any learning environment, including adult programming.

❑ Electronic technology is used not as a primary teaching tool but as a supplemental resource to reinforce or practice learning.

Did you know? Not all screens, media, or electronic technology are bad. However, they should not take the place of teacher interactions or teaching. For instance, children should be introduced to letters and their sounds through meaningful and personal experiences. Then they could use a computer game as one method of practicing using letters or playing with phonics. For more on developmentally appropriate uses of electronic technology, refer to the joint position statement released by the National Association for the Education of Young Children (NAEYC) and the Fred Rogers Center for Early Learning and Children's Media at Saint Vincent College at www.naeyc.org/files/naeyc/file/positions/PS_technology_WEB2.pdf.

❑ All media in the learning environment are free of advertising or branding.

PHYSICAL ACTIVITY ENVIRONMENT

Goal: The atmosphere and environment in our program support physical activity.

❑ Play equipment for physical activity is in good repair.

❑ Spaces provided for physical activity are safe.

❑ Spaces provided for physical activity are interesting and engaging to children.

Did you know? While a patchy field with one torn soccer net and no shade is technically a space for physical activity, it is not engaging or interesting to children. Spaces for physical activity should receive as much attention as other learning areas. Shady areas, lots of equipment in good repair, and natural features like trees and flowers are some of the things that make a space for physical play engaging.

❑ Teachers offer to children and ensure access to water before, during, and after physical activity (children under six months should receive extra breast milk or formula rather than water).

Section 7

Program Approach to Physical Activity

Most children are naturally physically active. They seem to have an endless supply of energy and prefer to run whenever they can, climb everything, and play active games with abandon. That natural instinct can quickly be lost if children are not exposed to ongoing opportunities and models for active lifestyles. Unfortunately, that can happen for many reasons. Here is a sampling:

- People have fewer reasons to be active. Many jobs require minimal manual labor. Fewer people farm food. Transportation is readily available. More **sedentary** leisure options, such as video games and computer activities, are available. This is true for adults as well as children.

- Some neighborhoods have few, if any, safe active play spaces for children.

- Children's physical activities are becoming more and more scheduled instead of happening naturally. For example, children attend adult-led baseball practice or go to tot-gymnastics classes instead of meeting at the neighborhood park for an unscheduled game or playing in the backyard sandbox. This matters because organized sports impose rules on children and make right/wrong judgments, eliminating opportunities to play creatively, freely, and spontaneously. (Participation in sports can be a largely positive experience for children, as long as it is age appropriate and not the only form of physical activity a child engages in.)

The goal of **physical activity** for children isn't to achieve a specific physical appearance or to be as strong or fast as someone else. In early childhood, balance, muscle and bone strength, coordination, and other motor skills are the underlying objectives associated with physical activity. The ultimate goal is to help children develop habits that will nurture lifelong, active lifestyles. They will do this best when the adults around them model and teach them how to build these important foundational habits and attitudes. Adults should help children learn to enjoy and value physical activity rather than treat it as a chore or competition. Building these attitudes and habits in early childhood increases the likelihood of children remaining physically active into adulthood. By promoting physical activity, you help children minimize their risk for many illnesses and injuries. You increase their chances of leading positive and active lives. The adults in children's lives should consciously teach and model positive body image and eliminate all references to unrealistic body images.

This section will address:

- Modeling and teaching positive behaviors and attitudes toward physical fitness: Children often learn from observing the adults around them. Knowing how to model and teach physical activity and fitness throughout the day can make a big impression on young learners.

- Program education: Educating children about physical activity and fitness requires some knowledge and understanding. There are many ways to enhance your curriculum with meaningful physical activity and fitness experiences.

Modeling and Teaching Positive Behaviors and Attitudes toward Physical Fitness

Children learn from what they see and experience throughout the day. When you model and teach healthy attitudes to physical activity, children will adopt these for themselves. You cannot simply tell children what they should be doing and not model it yourself. Of course, most children are naturally inclined to run freely, climb trees, and engage in other daily physical activity. But some children need to be prompted. Many adults have physical limitations that restrict their mobility. Regardless, being positive about physical activity, valuing its importance, and engaging in it to the best of your ability are more powerful than anything you could tell a child to do.

TEACHER MODELING BEHAVIORS

Goal: Teachers consistently model positive behaviors and attitudes toward physical activity and fitness. They encourage children to develop the same attitudes and behaviors.

❑ Teachers use positive language and engage in positive conversation about physical activity.

❑ Physical appearance or losing weight is never the focus of a physical activity.

❑ Teachers do not participate in or allow stereotyping, teasing, or other types of demeaning comments about body image or physical abilities.

Did you know? Negative and often unintentional comments about a person's physical appearance occur frequently. Have you ever told children that their chubby cheeks are so cute? Or watched children leave peers out of a game because they couldn't run fast enough? These are subtle but harmful forms of stereotyping. Allowing a child to discriminate against others because of their physical appearance or ability fosters the development of unconscious stereotypes and biases. Being the recipient of such comments hurts a child's self-esteem.

❑ Teachers engage in physical activity with the children during each physical activity period.

❑ Teachers are dressed so they can comfortably participate in physical activity with the children (for example, in tennis shoes and loose clothing).

❑ Teachers model enthusiasm and enjoyment during physical activity.

❑ Teachers speak about physical activity and outdoor environments positively.

Did you know? It's easy to let slip a negative comment like "I am so tired today, I do not feel like playing outside," or "Be careful, there are lots of hazards out here." These small statements can send big messages to children. Try modeling positive thoughts, such as "I sure am tired, but I know getting outside will give me energy," and "There are things to be careful of outside, but it is safe for us to play. We just need to pay attention."

TEACHING STRATEGIES AND INTERACTIONS

Goal: In our program, children participate in planned learning opportunities that emphasize physical activity.

❑ Teachers include opportunities for physical development throughout the day.

Did you know? Physical activity can happen all day long, not only during blocks of scheduled time. Play Simon Says during **transitions**. Practice measurement by measuring how far children jump. Practice child-friendly yoga while children are moving into rest time.

❑ Teachers focus on many aspects of physical development in their teaching, such as flexibility, coordination, balance, muscle strength, and agility.

❑ Teachers focus on relevant behavioral competencies, such as goal setting, self-assessment, physical confidence, and self-control when planning physical activities.

Did you know? If you are interested in physical development and related behavioral competencies, you can find many resources, including those listed in the additional resources section of this book, beginning on page 251.

❑ Children are never excluded from physical activity for any reason.

❑ Boys and girls have equal opportunities to participate in all types of physical and active play.

❑ Children of varied abilities are given equal chances to participate in all types of physical and active play.

❑ Program rules and providers' interactions do not inhibit physical activity. Instead, they ensure that play is safe and appropriate.

❑ Teachers acknowledge children's efforts at physical activity rather than their achievements.

❑ Teachers **scaffold** children's individual physical development. They include physical development goals in their lesson plans and conferences.

❑ Teachers are respectful of all people in their messages about body image.

Program Education

In child care, physical education is often minimal. It simply isn't a primary focus in early childhood. Granted, licensing and accreditation standards require specific amounts of time for physical activity and time outside. But there are few, if any, regulations addressing the teaching of physical activity and fitness. The assumption is that physical education develops naturally through active play. In fact, much of it does, but children can further benefit from specific teaching about physical activity and fitness. For these lessons to positively influence children's development and life choices, they must be taught throughout the day. As one of the primary domains, physical development requires more focus than it often receives. All physical development can't occur during activities like outdoor free play or children's activity CDs. While these are effective activities, you also need a deliberate focus on using physical activity to develop specific skills and abilities.

THE INDOOR LEARNING ENVIRONMENT

Goal: Our indoor learning environments promote physical activity.

❑ Each indoor learning environment (or classroom) has a space designated for active play.

❑ Physical development equipment, such as climbers, slides, or balance beams, is present in each learning environment.

❑ The learning environment includes displays, such as posters and books, that promote healthy habits.

❑ Portable active play materials, such as ribbons, balls, and parachutes, are readily available and used indoors every week.

Bonus Checklist

❑ The program has an indoor room dedicated to large-muscle play and activity.

THE OUTDOOR LEARNING ENVIRONMENT

Goal: Our outdoor physical environment promotes physical activity.

❑ The program has enough tricycles or other wheeled toys in good condition.

Did you know? Most states do not require helmets, but they are a good idea for children riding tricycles. This simple precaution can teach children an important, lifelong safety lesson.

❑ The outdoor environment includes a variety of fixed equipment that encourages active play.

❑ The outdoor space includes open play areas for activities involving movement or running.

❑ Sunscreen is applied daily in warm weather.

> **Did you know?** Sunscreen should be labeled *broad spectrum* with a sun protection factor (SPF) of at least fifteen, but preferably thirty or higher. It should be used according to the manufacturer's directions. It should be applied at least fifteen minutes before exposure to sun and reapplied every two hours or after a child becomes wet. Make sure sunscreen has not expired.

❑ The outdoor environment is free from hazards, is safe for play, and includes shaded areas.

> **Did you know?** If state licensing regulations do not address playground and/or outdoor safety or you need more information on the topic, refer to the US Consumer Product Safety Commission at http://www.cpsc.gov/cpscpub/pubs/playpubs.html.

❑ Children play outdoors every day except when the weather poses a significant health risk.

❑ Children are dressed appropriately for the weather and are allowed to regulate their own need for more or less warm clothing, such as jackets and hats.

❑ Extra clothing is available to supplement children's own.

> **Did you know?** Children should go outside every day, except when weather poses a significant health risk. This means that even if it is chillier or warmer than usual, children should still go outside. Families should be required to bring extra clothes, appropriate shoes, sunscreen, sun hats, and other necessary supplies. Programs should have extra supplies on hand in case families forget something. In mild climates, it is easy to be caught off guard by sudden changes in the weather. Prepare for these days so children don't miss out on physical play and new experiences.

LEARNING ACTIVITIES

Goal: The daily lesson plans, curriculum, and/or children's activities consistently focus on physical activity and fitness.

❑ Physical activity is part of the daily lesson plan.

❑ Children engage in **vigorous activity**, such as running, dancing, or skipping, every day. (See appendix F in this book to review examples of vigorous and moderate activities for young children.)

❑ Physical activities are rotated or changed often to ensure children experience variety and can find activities they enjoy. (See appendix F to review examples of vigorous and moderate activities for young children.)

❑ Physical activity times include both free play and **structured,** or **planned,** activities every day.

❑ Children are not required to participate in all physical activity, but they are always invited and encouraged.

❑ The program modifies physical activities for individual children as needed.

❑ Walking field trips and/or field trips to places where physical activity occurs are part of the program.

❑ Physical activities are noncompetitive and inclusive. All children have equal playtime and enjoyment.

❑ The weekly lesson plan includes:

   ❑ stretching activities, such as child-appropriate yoga
   ❑ balance and coordination activities or games, such as Simon Says
   ❑ dance or other creative movement

Bonus Checklist

❑ A research-based physical activity curriculum is used as a resource or guide.

Did you know? Many physical activity and fitness curricula are available for young children. Some of these curricula also address other aspects of healthy development, such as nutrition. A program doesn't need to follow the curriculum exactly, but it is important to use reliable and developmentally appropriate resources.

❑ The program is involved in fitness-related community activities, such as a walk for hunger, a jump-rope-athon, a walk-or-bike-to-work day, or a family health day.

❑ The program offers education or workshops on positive parenting during physical activities, such as MNPlays http://www.cehd.umn.edu/MNYSRC/programs/mnplays.html.

❑ The program supports community initiatives related to physical activity, such as safe bike paths, renovations on a community swimming pool, or park cleanup initiatives.

INFANTS' PHYSICAL ACTIVITY

Goal: Daily lesson plans, curriculum, and activities offered to infants include developmentally appropriate physical experiences.

❑ Infants have at least two outdoor experiences per day (only one can be a buggy or stroller ride). Infants in part-day programs need at least one experience.

❑ Physical activities for infants promote exploring their environment.

❑ Infants' spaces are safe for movement and exploration.

❑ Infants spend less than ten minutes at a time in restraining devices that limit free movement, such as swings, bouncy seats, and exersaucers. No children spend more than thirty minutes per day in a restraining device.

Did you know? The term *restraining device* refers to things like swings, exersaucers, and bouncy seats—devices in which infants are buckled and therefore restrained. While family members may choose to use these at home, you should limit or eliminate their use in your program. They do not contribute to a child's development and in some cases can impede it if they are overused. Infants miss out on important muscle development time when they are in restraining devices.

❑ Structured activities that support infants' development are planned daily. These include tummy time, hand-eye coordination, crawling practice, reaching for an object, and grasping an item intentionally. (See appendix B to review recommended physical activity guidelines for infants.)

❑ Infants remain in cribs only while they are sleeping.

TODDLERS' PHYSICAL ACTIVITY

Goal: The daily lesson plans, curriculum, and activities offered to toddlers include developmentally appropriate physical experiences.

❑ A minimum of sixty minutes per day is allotted for **unstructured** physical activity for toddlers. This time does not have to be consecutive. For toddlers in half-day programs, only thirty minutes per day is needed.

❏ A minimum of thirty minutes per day is allotted for structured physical activity for toddlers. This time does not have to be consecutive. For toddlers in half-day programs, only fifteen minutes are needed.

❏ Toddlers do not spend more than fifteen minutes at a time in a group or a teacher-led **sedentary** activity except naptime or mealtime.

❏ Structured physical activities for toddlers support the development of movement skills. These, in turn, serve as the foundations for more complex skills. For example, toddlers can work on jumping, which leads to dexterity, coordination, and bone strength. (See appendix B to review recommended physical activity guidelines for toddlers.)

❏ Toddlers' spaces are safe for movement and exploration.

PRESCHOOLERS' PHYSICAL ACTIVITY

Goal: The daily lesson plans, curriculum, and activities offered to preschoolers include developmentally appropriate physical experiences.

❏ A minimum of sixty minutes per day is allotted for unstructured physical activity for preschoolers. These do not have to be consecutive. Those in half-day programs need only thirty minutes.

❏ A minimum of sixty minutes per day is allotted for structured activity for preschoolers. These do not have to be consecutive. Those in half-day programs need only thirty minutes.

❏ Preschoolers do not spend more than twenty minutes in a group or teacher-led sedentary activity except naptime or mealtime.

❏ Structured physical activities for preschoolers support the development of movement skills. These, in turn, serve as foundations for more complex skills. For example, preschoolers can play games with two- or three-step directions that support coordinating multiple skills and movements. (See appendix B to review recommended physical activity guidelines for preschoolers.)

❏ Preschoolers' spaces are safe for movement and exploration.

SCHOOLAGERS' PHYSICAL ACTIVITY

Goal: The daily lesson plans, curriculum, and activities offered to school-age children include developmentally appropriate physical experiences.

❑ A minimum of thirty minutes is allotted for unstructured physical activity for schoolagers who attend before- and after-school programs. Sixty minutes are allotted for schoolagers attending full-day programs. The time does not have to be consecutive.

❑ A minimum of thirty minutes is allotted for structured physical activity for schoolagers who attend before- and after-school programs. Sixty minutes are allotted for schoolagers attending full-day programs. The time does not have to be consecutive.

❑ Schoolagers do not spend more than thirty minutes in a group or teacher-led sedentary activity.

❑ Schoolagers' spaces are safe for movement and exploration.

Section 8

Physical Activity and Fitness Education and Resources for Families

Health and physical **fitness** can be sensitive topics. It is never your role to judge a family or to critique its choices. Children and families who do not have healthy, active lifestyles do not want to be unhealthy. It is more likely that they don't have access to resources, are overwhelmed by the array of available advice and information, or don't know how to turn what they've heard into practical steps for their family. If families lack the best information, how can they make the right choices for their children? Fortunately, many credible resources are available to families and early childhood professionals to guide decisions. Great resources are also available for children. You can help families by promoting opportunities, sharing reliable resources, and working in partnership to ensure the health and physical development of children.

Early childhood professionals focus on all types of child development. They—and you—are considered credible and trusted resources by families. **Physical activity** and fitness are a significant part of physical development, so they deserve your attention and that of families. Educators and coaches can help children with physical activity, but family members and parents remain significant influences on children's attitudes and behaviors. If your program offers reliable resources about physical activity and fitness, families are likely to be receptive to them.

This section will address:

- Family support: Providing resources and identifying community support for families related to physical activity and fitness helps ensure children have positive physical opportunities at home as well.

- Program resources: Making resources available to teachers related to physical activity and fitness will be useful for both teachers new to planning physical activity and those just looking for fresh ideas.

Family Support

Many families find it hard to fit physical activity and fitness into their busy routines. Add the nonstop advertisements and media reports about fitness trends, programs, and dangers of fitness products, and people can feel overwhelmed. When they're overwhelmed, they may stop before they even get started. Provide families with reliable and relevant information. Engage and support them in physical activity and fitness.

FAMILY SUPPORT

Goal: We share and promote physical activity and family fitness opportunities within our community of families.

❏ Our program newsletter includes a regular section dedicated to physical activity.

❏ We recognize family members' role as their child's primary role models and teachers. We work to develop partnerships with families to promote children's physical activity and fitness.

❏ We provide information on limiting screen time: why it's important and ways to do it effectively.

❏ We provide opportunities for families to become involved in our physical activity curriculum.

❏ We partner with community resources to promote physical activity and fitness.

❏ We share information and opportunities for families to engage in physical activity together.

❏ We provide resources to families about how to make physical activity experiences positive for young children.

❏ We inform families about local physical activity opportunities, such as a family 5K run/walk and discounted memberships at a fitness club.

Did you know? Community organizations that focus on physical activity and health welcome the chance to partner with child care programs. A local fitness center could host a program about physical activities. Instead of hosting an end-of-year cookout, you could host an end-of-year family day in a local park. You could invite college athletes to play with the children and share their enthusiasm for physical activity. Sharing information about community events can support families. Partnering with community programs doesn't have to be complicated or time-consuming; the programs will often appreciate the opportunity to connect with multiple families, while the families in your program can benefit. Check out the organization before bringing it into your program to be sure it's credible. You don't want its time with families to turn into a sales presentation.

Program Resources

Child care programs and teachers are viewed as trusted and reliable resources on child development by families. When families want to learn more about a topic related to their young children, they often look to you first. It's unlikely you will know every fact about every topic. But when you are familiar with current, reliable, resources, you can refer families to what they need to know when they need to know it.

PROGRAM RESOURCES

Goal: Our program has accurate and relevant resources about physical activity and fitness. Both families and teachers use these.

❑ Books, DVDs, and/or other resources on physical activity are available in our family lending library.

❑ Books, DVDs, and/or other resources on physical activity are available in our teacher resource library.

❑ The program provides resources for teachers to help them incorporate physical activity into their lesson plans.

❑ The program makes children's books about physical activity and fitness available to children.

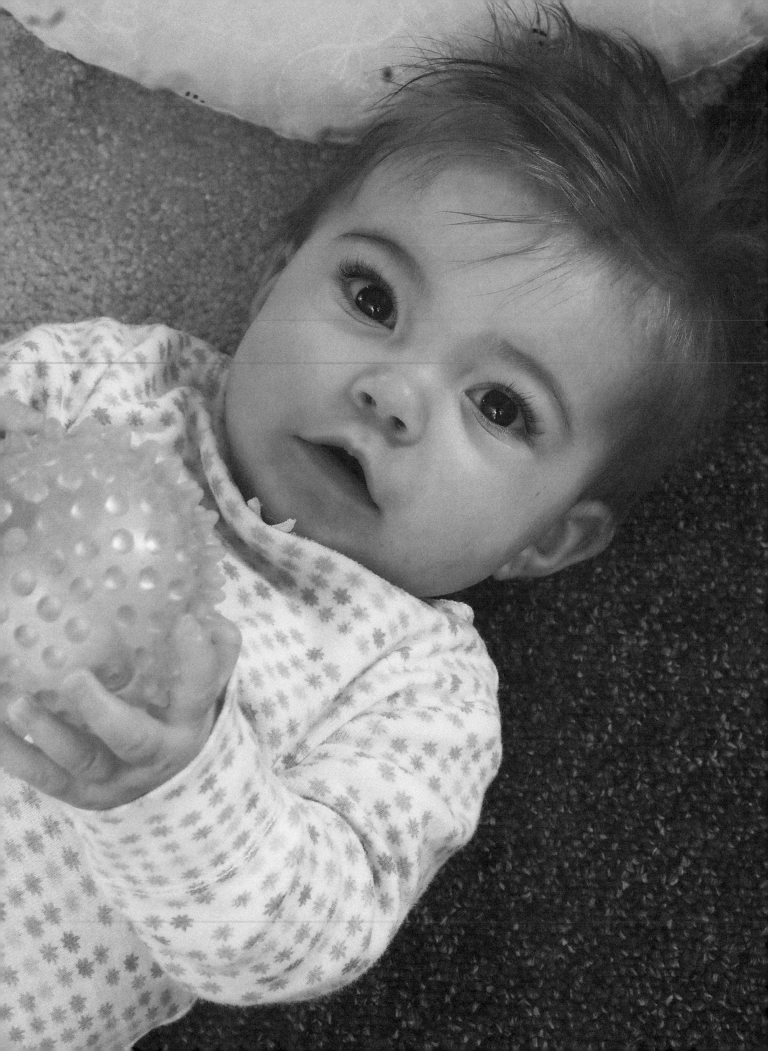

Part 3

Emotional Health and Resilience

When it comes to a child's overall healthy development, emotional health and **resilience** are as important as physical wellness and can equally impact the quality of a child's or adult's life. Terms such as *emotional health* and *mental wellness* often conjure up thoughts of cognitive disabilities, behavioral disorders, or issues such as depression or anxiety. While mental health issues like these are significant aspects of emotional health, they are outside the realm of this book. Instead, this part of the book focuses on strategies to nurture and enhance children's development in ways that contribute to their lifelong emotional health and wellness. If careful and intentional attention is given to developing and supporting emotional health and wellness, then not only will children have the skills they need to have rich and rewarding lives, but they may also avoid or minimize many future challenges. Essentially, part 3 of this book ensures teachers are able to support the creation of a social and emotional toolbox full of skills and abilities that will help children experience lifelong success in their personal, professional, and academic experiences.

The Challenge

Academics have gotten a lot of attention in the past decade. Our schools have become more and more focused on academic content, and many enrichments like music and recess have been minimized or eliminated. At the same time, children's learning and progress are tested, measured, and compared more than ever before, increasing the pressure to perform and demonstrate outcomes. Historically, this debate over the focus on academics was left to the primary and secondary educators. As pressure has mounted for growth and achievement that can be demonstrated on a test, families have turned up their expectations—expectations not always appropriate, but increased expectations nonetheless—for early childhood, and the focus on cognitive development over all other forms of development has oozed its way into our profession. This imbalance is neither developmentally appropriate for young children during childhood, nor does it support healthy long-term school and life success. Certainly math, science, and literacy are important areas of education, and children need skills in these areas to be successful. But social and emotional development deserve as much or even more attention. If children can solve complex calculations but can't control their emotions, their career and life satisfaction will be much lower. How will they someday succeed in the workplace if they can't develop peer relationships? How will they work on collaborative assignments in high school and college if they don't know how to share? Because many social-emotional skills can't be tested easily, their development is rarely measured.

In today's culture, the things that get measured are all that seem to matter. As an early childhood educator, you need to ensure that the care and learning in your program are based on what research indicates is best, rather than on social pressures. You must explain why in the early years your approach produces better results than more academic ones. It doesn't have to be an either-or situation. Children can enjoy development and learning in all domains: cognitive, physical, social, and emotional. The goal should be simply to prepare children for life, not just for kindergarten or school. You need to help them learn to develop successful relationships, enjoy career success, problem solve, make appropriate decisions, express themselves, and contribute to the world positively. As a publication of the Alliance for Childhood says, "Rather than standards, well-prepared early educators need appropriate guidelines they can apply with flexibility. Rather than testing narrow skills, we should broadly gauge cognitive, social-emotional, and physical areas, as well as creativity and other essential qualities of human life" (Almon and Miller 2011, 3).

What Is Emotional Health and Resilience?

Emotional health and resilience are overarching concepts that include development in the social and emotional domains, such as developing healthy relationships, communication skills, and emotional regulation, as well as other areas related to social and emotional development: **attachment**, positive **behavior guidance**, and **approaches to learning**. Together, these areas of development and experiences contribute to children's emotional health and resilience.

PROTECTIVE FACTORS

Researchers who study resilience spend a lot of time trying to identify what happens in young children's lives that protects them from difficult situations. Why do some children with an abusive parent succeed while others do not? Why does one teenager who loses a parent continue to thrive while another does not? Researchers have compared adults from equally difficult backgrounds who grew up in dangerous neighborhoods, went to poorly performing schools, and came from families with little or no money. Some of the people studied continued to do poorly as adults, while others did not. Some of these adults broke the cycle, went on to college, and achieved other successes. Researchers asked why some of these adults succeeded while others failed, when all had the same background. Studies demonstrated the existence of protective factors that made the difference. Protective factors are skills or abilities that protect a child or adult from the impact of risk factors. According to the Devereux Foundation, attachment to caring adults, personal initiative, and ability to express and control emotions are the most critical protective factors. For example, a secure attachment protects a child who is faced with a personal challenge. Personal initiative helps a child who struggles with learning a new skill to keep trying and not give up. The ability to express and control emotions protects a child from making impulsive decisions based on difficult emotions.

FAMILY INVOLVEMENT

Family support and involvement are significant factors of emotional health and **resilience**. Parents, family members, and you should work together to support a child. The often-used phrase "It takes a village to raise a child" is true in many ways. You should not compartmentalize care and support for a child. You must weave your efforts together to provide the most support, guidance, and love you can offer to each child. Many parents and family members have wonderful natural abilities and instincts for raising children (they must have had good social-emotional development when they were children!). Others lack these abilities and instincts. They actually hinder or harm their children's development. Those children need your intervention. Professionals in the field of early childhood education have information and insights that the average family member does not. Working together, you and families can harmoniously provide the best childhood experiences possible. Most families want to do what's best for their children. They will eagerly improve their skills or change their approach if they have the opportunity. If they receive informed, nonjudgmental support from you, they are very likely to respond in positive ways.

Why Is Resilience Important?

Resilience is the ability to bounce back after coping with adversity or challenges. This can be disappointment about a block tower falling down, managing the frustration of not getting a turn, or adapting to parents' divorce. Resilience skills don't guarantee that life events won't have a lasting or negative impact, but they do significantly increase the chance that a person can overcome adversity. As Sesame Workshop maintains, "Developing effective resilience skills to cope with stressful situations at early stages in children's development can have a significant impact on children's well-being and their future success in all areas of life" (Sesame Street Child Resilience Initiative 2011, 3).

Children are indeed born with basic resilience skills. These skills help them try and try again, all day long. But without support and nurturing, these skills can fade. All children need resilience skills; in many ways, these skills serve as coats of armor. We hope children won't suffer or endure difficult life events, such as the death of a loved one, loss of a home, abuse, lack of food, or other hardships that pose significant challenges. The future challenges that children in your care will face are unclear. Supporting their existing skills and helping them develop further can prepare and protect children from many life situations. Helping them learn these skills can minimize the damage difficult life situations can do. Child psychologist Ann Masten says, "The great surprise of resilience research is the ordinariness of the phenomena. Resilience appears to be a common phenomenon that results in most cases from the operation of basic human adaptational systems. If those systems are protected and in good working order, development is robust even in the face of severe adversity; if these major systems are impaired . . . then the risk for developmental problems is much greater" (2001, 227).

What Should the Early Care and Education Community Do?

The early childhood education community can do a lot to support the children in care and increase their emotional health and resilience. Understanding the value of a child's emotional health and development is the first step. Prioritizing social and emotional development and communicating its value to parents, families, and the community is the second step. As Masten says, "The great threats to human development are those that jeopardize the systems underlying these adaptive processes, including brain development and cognition, caregiver–child relationships, regulation of emotion and behavior, and the motivation for learning and engaging in the environment" (2001, 234).

Early childhood professionals can avoid threats to children's emotional health and resilience and support the development of adaptive systems. Doing so requires patience and recognition that opportunities occur in small moments every day. When children are eagerly welcomed in the morning, allowed to problem solve when their first attempts fail, and supported while they work out a conflict with a peer, they develop important social-emotional skills, and they also build resilience. When you intentionally support this development, children thrive.

Note: Early childhood educators and providers should never diagnose, treat, or attempt to heal serious mental health problems. It is important to report any signs of serious emotional or mental health challenges to appropriate authorities right away.

Section 9

Sociability

Sociability is the *ability* to engage successfully in *social* experiences. Social skills are essential to success in life and school. According to Bear and Watkins, they often function as gatekeepers, providing (or denying) children important social experiences. These, in turn, lead to further developmental opportunities, such as effective communication abilities, relationship skills like compromise and perspective taking, development of a positive sense of self, and even increased academic success. Research consistently demonstrates links between social-emotional skills and academic achievement in primary and secondary grades (quoted in Durlak et al. 2011). Children who don't develop these important skills miss out on important developmental opportunities. George Vaillant, director of one of the most comprehensive longitudinal studies in history, said, "It is social aptitude, not intellectual brilliance or parental social class, that leads to successful aging" (quoted in Shenk 2009).

Children's instinctual social skills are influenced by their **temperament**, that of the adults who care for them, the context in which they live, and their relationships with caregivers. These combined influences can strongly affect children's sociability. Beyond developing strong **attachments**, children's other early social skills must be nurtured, supported, and expanded upon. Fortunately, support can occur through simple, daily interactions and social experiences. Mastery of these skills is the long-term goal.

Child care programs must ensure that all children have equal opportunities to learn and practice social skills in a supportive environment. Whatever their attachment to **primary caregivers**, home and cultural life, or temperament, they need practice in these skills. Social skills affect all aspects of children's growth, development, and health. These should be a priority in your program.

This section will address:

- Attachment: Attachment is arguably the most significant social-emotional experience in a young child's life. The quality of a child's early attachments can have impact now and in the future. Daily practices that support, develop, and maintain attachments with parents and teachers are crucial components of a supportive early childhood program.

- Developing healthy relationships: Children who can develop positive relationships with adults and peers that include give and take, negotiation, problem-solving, empathy, and other important relationship skills have better outcomes in multiple areas, from school to life satisfaction.

- Communication skills: Communication skills are important for school and life success. Techniques that nurture effective communication skills can be implemented from infancy.

Attachment

One of the first social and emotional milestones in a child's life, and perhaps the most critical, is developing an **attachment** to adults. Attachment can be thought of as the sense of safety and security a child feels from an adult. Children's first relationships with parents and caregivers are so critical to their wellness and development that they can't be overstated. Developing a trusting, unconditionally loving connection with consistent caregivers is the foundation for all other development. A child without a positive attachment early in life is akin to a house built without a foundation. Attachments influence children's view of the world, the quality of their relationships, their academic achievement, even their brain development. Ideally, children form positive attachments to parents, other family members, and caregivers (including early childhood teachers). If they do not develop attachments to parents or other consistent family members, it becomes even more essential that they develop these attachments with you.

Most children in child care have developed strong attachments with their parent (or other adults primarily responsible for the child's care) at home. Early care and education programs should support the development of secondary (or primary) attachments between child and teacher as well: "The deeper a child's trust in the loving quality and security of your caregiving, the more likely the child will form a secure attachment with the teacher or caregiver" (Honig 2010, 26). Continuous discussion and debate exist on the value and impact of a child's early attachments. Some take a fatalistic view and doom those with poor early attachments to a lifetime of challenges. Others do not consider early attachments the only opportunities for positive paths in life. Attachment theorists and researchers agree that children's first attachments are important and shape much of their future: "It is safe to say that although many variables affect lifespan development, babies' first relationships are among the most important, and attachment is the reason for this" (Mooney 2010, 7). Children who are attached to one or more adults in their lives are more confident, more willing to explore and experiment, more trusting, and very often exhibit fewer challenging behaviors. You should ensure that children form strong attachments early in life so they can grow and thrive.

SUPPORTING PARENT-CHILD ATTACHMENT

Goal: To the extent possible, we support the development and maintenance of a positive, warm, consistent relationship between parent and child.

❑ Teachers understand and support parents as children's primary caregivers and teachers.

❑ Teachers help parents and children develop supportive and positive drop-off and pickup routines.

❑ Teachers do not allow parents to sneak out or otherwise trick their children.

❑ Teachers ensure they have time to listen to parents, answer their questions, and empathize with their challenges.

❑ Teachers help parents understand developmentally appropriate behaviors and expectations that may be challenging them.

❑ Teachers are attentive to interactions between parents and children and are prepared to intervene if the interactions are harmful.

Did you know? While some interactions between parent and child may be negative, most of them are not harmful. Children cry because they don't want to clean up, or have a tantrum because their parents pick them up in the middle of a fun activity. These are par for the course in a child care program. But some interactions can be harmful. Perhaps a parent spanks a child or threatens physical abuse in your facility. Maybe the parents smell like alcohol when they pick their children up, or they are verbally abusive, calling the child "stupid" or claiming they won't love him if he isn't "good." Maybe the parents just look overwhelmed and can't respond to typical yet challenging children's behavior. You must be alert to situations like these. Helping parents connect with resources or involving a third party, like child protection services, might make a world of difference to the child and the child-parent relationship. It is not easy, but it is important.

SUPPORTING TEACHER-CHILD ATTACHMENT

Goal: Teachers in our program purposefully develop secure attachments with the children in their care.

❑ Children have the same teacher for at least a full year when possible.

❑ Children are in the same care and learning environment (classroom) for at least a year.

❑ Teachers' schedules and responsibilities are developed to maximize time with the children in their care.

❑ When more than one teacher shares a learning environment, children are assigned to a primary caregiver.

❑ If a teacher has to be absent, children are told immediately, and they can express their feelings and ask questions.

❑ If a teacher leaves the program, children can express their feelings and ask questions.

Did you know? Children don't always verbally express their concern or distress when you are absent or unavailable. They certainly do feel it and may even express their feelings through behavior. Adults easily understand the reasons for absences or changes in schedule. Children do not. In fact, inconsistency or change in teachers can disrupt children's learning and progress. If you show up late or miss work, you may not mean to affect children, but your behavior certainly does. Consistency is important. Of course, things happen and schedules change, but it is important to understand the impact and minimize disruption as much as possible.

❑ Teachers are positive and consistent in their mood, behavior, and affection for all children.

❑ Teachers refrain from teasing, sarcasm, irony, and other verbal communication that may be hard for children to interpret.

❑ Teachers demonstrate affection that meets each child's needs and is culturally appropriate.

❑ Teachers use consistent and soothing comfort strategies, individualized for the needs of each child.

❑ To minimize anxiety and fear, people unknown to infants and toddlers are rarely allowed in infant/toddler environments.

❑ Teachers respond to and reassure all children who exhibit signs of distress.

Bonus Checklist

❑ Children have the same teacher for two years or more.

DAILY TRANSITIONS

Goal: Transitions are minimal and are smooth and gradual.

❑ Transitions during the day are smooth, gradual, and include warnings.

❑ Individual children are assisted with transitions as needed.

❑ Individual needs of children are considered during transitions.

❑ Transitions are used as learning opportunities.

❑ Children are not shifted between classrooms throughout the day (centers only).

TRANSITIONS WITHIN THE PROGRAM

Goal: Transitions within the program are emotionally supportive, developmentally appropriate, and meet individual children's needs.

❏ If children transition to a new care environment or classroom, they have the opportunity to
  ❏ gradually make the transition over at least two weeks
  ❏ bring a comfort item as needed
  ❏ visit the new environment with their current teacher
  ❏ transition when they are developmentally ready

Did you know? It is tempting to move children on the basis of birth dates, specific months, or mastery of a certain skill, like being able to use the toilet independently. These approaches do not consider children's overall developmental needs. It is best to move children on when they demonstrate cognitive, physical, social, and emotional readiness to advance. This may require revising your transition policies or buying diapering equipment for a preschool environment.

❏ When children transition to another learning environment (classroom), every effort is made to move them with at least one other familiar child.

❏ When children are scheduled to transition, their families are notified and the transition plan is discussed in detail. Family members and children can express feelings and ask questions.

Bonus Checklist

❏ If children change learning environments (classrooms), their teacher continues with them for at least two years.

TRANSITIONS OUTSIDE THE PROGRAM

Goal: The program supports children when they transition into new learning environments away from the program.

❏ When children transition to kindergarten, their teacher(s) work with the kindergarten teacher and/or school to understand how to best prepare them.

❏ Children are encouraged to express their feelings and ask questions about changing programs or schools. Preparation for changing programs includes reading stories to the children about the transition and providing opportunities for dramatic play to practice.

Developing Healthy Relationships

"Good relationships are key to effective teaching and guidance in social, emotional, and behavioral development" (Fox et al. 2003). Children and adults learn about themselves and develop social-emotional skills through relationships. Besides developing healthy attachments to parents and other adult caregivers, young children need to develop peer relationships or friendships. This is a primary task for young children and becomes increasingly significant throughout childhood and adolescence. Children benefit in many ways from strong, reliable, and supportive friendships, just as they do from early attachments to adults.

When you focus on developing children's social skills from their earliest moments, you are spending your time wisely. Negotiating, perspective taking, compromising, sharing, problem solving, and developing **empathy** are essential life skills that develop as children build and develop relationships. According to Lise Fox, an expert in child behavior, "In the context of supportive relationships, children develop positive self-concept, confidence, and a sense of safety that help reduce the occurrence of challenging behavior. As such, the time spent building a strong relationship is probably less than the time required to implement more elaborate and time-consuming strategies" (Fox et al. 2003). Just imagine adults who don't have the ability to share, take turns, or compromise trying to succeed in a typical office job. They would have a difficult time even if they were competent at their tasks. People can change and learn throughout life, but early childhood patterns of good peer relationships are fairly strong predictors of children's future competence or deviance (National Research Council and Institute of Medicine 2000).

The value of these first relationships cannot be overstated. A positive relationship with teachers functions as a home base and security blanket—it makes learning, exploration, experimentation, and engagement possible. These first relationships influence how children feel about themselves and others, about learning and teachers, and about peer relationships (Kersey and Masterson 2011). In the words of early childhood experts, "Every interaction with you is an opportunity for children to develop positive feelings about themselves" (Willis and Schiller 2011, 13).

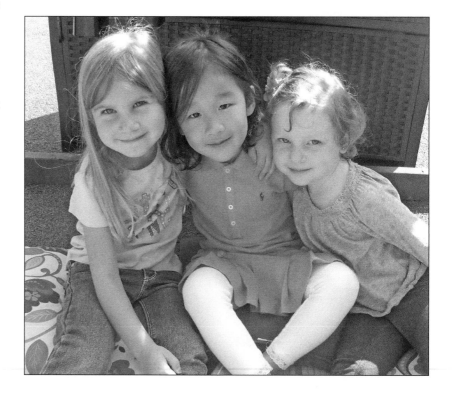

PROSOCIAL BEHAVIOR

Goal: The children in the program have many opportunities to develop age-appropriate prosocial behaviors.

❑ Teachers express joy when each child arrives for the day.

❑ Teachers express kindness when entering into play or other activities with children.

❑ Teachers interact at eye level with children.

❑ Teachers model, teach, and encourage the use of verbal manners, such as "Please," "Thank you," and "Excuse me."

❑ Teachers teach and model social norms, such as taking turns during conversation, "listening" to body language, and respecting physical space.

❑ Teachers model and teach respect for others' opinions, perspectives, feelings, and ideas.

❑ Teachers model and teach **sympathy** and **empathy**.

Did you know? Opportunities to model and teach sympathy and empathy happen every day. You can give voice to children's actions so they can learn from them. For instance, you might say, "I see Joshua sitting by himself. I wonder if he is feeling lonely. I am going to go check on him to make sure he is feeling okay." You can use props like puppets, books, toy animals, felt board stories, and dolls to act out scenarios. You can acknowledge children's emerging efforts to care for each other. Even an infant can demonstrate empathy by crying at the sound of another infant's cries. Children as young as eighteen months can show signs of compassion by giving a crying child their comfort items. The capacity for empathy and sympathy already exists in each child. It's up to you to nurture those instincts in children.

❑ Teachers model and teach treating children equally. They meet individual needs, including gender, ethnicity, religion, and ability.

❑ Teachers plan opportunities for children to learn and practice
    ❑ cooperation
    ❑ negotiation
    ❑ compromise
    ❑ problem solving
    ❑ sharing
    ❑ expression of desires or ideas
    ❑ empathy

❏ The environment and materials foster prosocial behavior, such as cooperation and group work.

PEER RELATIONSHIPS

Goal: Teachers understand the value of peer relationships. They support and promote the development of children's relationship skills and friendships.

❏ Teachers understand the stages of play and have appropriate expectations for children's behavior.

❏ Teachers promote understanding of others' perspectives.

Did you know? We've all heard or asked the question, "How would that make you feel?" Many children don't know how to answer this question. They haven't yet developed their ability to consider another person's perspective. Talk about perspective during dramatic play or while you read stories. Doing so promotes development of this skill.

❏ When children argue or fight, teachers help them learn conflict resolution skills rather than finding fault or blaming.

❏ Teachers help children enter play situations when they need assistance.

❏ The environment provides places for pairs or small groups of children to work well together.

❏ Teachers do not engage in or tolerate teasing or bullying.

❏ Teachers model and teach sharing. They do not expect children to always share, and they take into account each child's age, developmental stage, and situation.

Did you know? Sharing isn't always appropriate. In fact, until they are about three years old, sharing is a concept most children cannot grasp and find very distressing. Once they understand it, sharing isn't always appropriate. For example, Josephina patiently waits her turn to play with the grocery cart. After she has played with it a few minutes, Devyn tries to take it from her. Ms. Nancy notices the conflict and says, "Share, you two." This is unfair to Josephina, who demonstrated good self-regulation by waiting her turn. Devyn doesn't learn the social skills she needs to get what she wants. Ms. Nancy's instruction to share hasn't helped anyone. In other situations, sharing may be the right thing to teach and expect. You should consider each child and each situation individually before expecting children to share.

❑ Teachers plan opportunities for age-appropriate, individual, and small- and large-group activities throughout each day.

❑ Teachers use small-group time so children can practice social skills with their peers.

RELATIONSHIPS WITH ADULTS

Goal: Teachers nurture and support development of adult-child relationships.

❑ Teachers are genuinely interested in and respect children's ideas, feelings, opinions, perspectives, and conversations.

❑ Teachers provide plentiful opportunities for child-led conversations.

❑ Teachers keep their promises to children.

Did you know? Keeping promises to children is simple to do and part of your daily interactions. If you say you'll give a child a turn, then you should give that child a turn. If you say you'll be right back, then you should be right back. Of course, sometimes a promise can't be fulfilled. Maybe parents pick a child up before he gets his turn. You need to address such changes in plan and explain why they occurred. These everyday opportunities reinforce trust between children and you and help children feel safe in their environment.

❑ If unexpected changes in routines or planned activities occur, you explain why and what will happen instead.

❑ Teachers are available to listen to or reassure children and do not dismiss their concerns.

Did you know? When you say, "You're okay, you're okay," to crying infants, the infants—if they could talk—would likely say, "Can you see me crying my eyes out here? I am clearly NOT okay." Instead, you can assure children that they will be okay, that you are there to take care of them, or that what they are worried about isn't going to happen. Saying, "You're okay," "You're fine," or "There's nothing to cry about" dismisses children's feelings and often contributes to increased concern, worry, or anxiety.

❑ Teachers are consistent in their emotions, behaviors, and expectations.

Did you know? Showing up to care for children grumpy, tired, or preoccupied by your own worries has an impact on children. If your moods are up, down, or unpredictable, children can't connect or build trust. It is a big responsibility, but no matter what happens outside of the program, you must be 100 percent emotionally consistent and present for the children in your care.

❑ Teachers express unconditional kindness and respect for all children in their care.

Communication Skills

Communication skills are both simple and complex. They include the first sounds and expressions infants make, as well as the nuanced tones and body language used often in conversations. Communication skills include the ability to express oneself through words and to accurately interpret what others are expressing. Children should learn from an early age that words have value and meaning. They need to understand that listening is as important as speaking and that communicating through words is an essential life tool. Janellen Huttenlocher reinforces this idea in *Mind in the Making* (as quoted in Galinsky 2010, 141): "Everything children are going to learn, they are going to learn through their ability to understand language and to produce language."

From their first attempts at communication, children are learning how, when, and why to use their communication skills. How adults respond to them helps children understand verbal communication and its uses. As they continue to grow and develop, their communication skills become increasingly complex and important. You must support this development.

EMERGING COMMUNICATION

Goal: In our program, we nurture and support children's preverbal and emerging communication skills.

❑ When speaking with infants, teachers make eye contact.

❑ When speaking with infants, teachers use conventional language rather than baby talk.

❑ Teachers respond to children's preverbal attempts to communicate verbally and through body language.

❑ Teachers have conversations with preverbal children, pausing occasionally to allow children to respond.

❑ Teachers use routine times as opportunities for one-on-one conversations with preverbal children.

❑ Teachers help preverbal children find the words to describe and/or extend their thoughts.

❑ Teachers ensure all children are read aloud to at least twice a day (at least once a day in half-day programs).

❑ Teachers use expressive and varied language.

❑ Teachers use words that are familiar and new to preverbal children.

❑ Teachers use different tones of voice consistent with their own emotions when speaking to preverbal children.

COMMUNICATION SKILLS

Goal: Through our interactions with children, we support the development of language and communication skills.

❑ Teachers use new and familiar words with children.

❑ Teachers model and teach **receptive/active listening**.

❑ Teachers help children analyze the meaning or intent behind communication.

❑ Teachers translate their and children's thoughts into writing each day.

❑ Teachers use **conversational language** with children more often than **directive language**.

❑ Teachers do not use rhetorical phrases like, "How many times do I have to tell you . . . ?" or "Didn't I just say . . . ?"

❑ Teachers do not use sarcasm or irony when speaking to or around children.

❑ Teachers model respectful, reciprocal conversations with other adults in front of children.

Did you know? Those little ears can pick up everything. Children aren't likely to understand parts of adult conversations. But they'll make meaning out of them anyway. For instance, a little boy in a military family started crying while waiting for his mother to take him home. His mother was talking to his teacher and said, "It seems like this war is never going to end, and Jim will never come home." Jim was the little boy's father. Although Jim was coming home soon, the boy took his mother's statement literally. Be careful when speaking in front of children. Don't hesitate to ask a parent to stop or pause if the conversation is not appropriate for little listeners.

❑ Teachers use appropriate body language when speaking with or near children.

❑ Teachers use appropriate language and grammar.

❑ Teachers build children's vocabularies.

❑ Teachers give children their full attention during conversations.

❑ When teachers converse with children, they pause occasionally to allow children to respond.

❑ Teachers use descriptive and varied language.

❑ Children can practice conversing, including listening and taking turns speaking.

❑ Teachers help children practice expressing themselves. They help them develop vocabularies that allow them expression.

Did you know? Imagine you're driving down a road, and another driver suddenly cuts you off and nearly causes an accident. If I asked you to use your words, what would you say? *Use your words* has become an overused phrase with good intentions behind it. If you tell children "use your words," be certain they know emotionally expressive words and can attach those to their feelings.

❑ Teachers consider the cultural or developmental nuances of children's communication skills and modify their conversations and interactions with individual children appropriately.

Did you know? Some children live in families that do not value emotional expression. In other families, children are not expected to speak unless spoken to. Such children will have different communication skills and approaches than children from expressive and highly communicative families. Children coping with developmental challenges or delays also have different communication abilities. Adapt your expectations to each child.

Section 10

Emotional Intelligence

Howard Gardener first introduced the idea of multiple intelligences in 1983. His theory proposed that intelligence was not simply a measure of cognitive knowledge. A person could have intelligence in other areas such as music, spatial/visual, or linguistics. Gardener's theory asserts that the question to ask is not, How smart is this child? but How is this child smart? While debate continues on Gardener's definitions of intelligence and his theory in general, he opened the door to thinking about a range of intelligence.

The concept of **emotional intelligence** has been around since the early twentieth century. Many scientists and psychologists have stated that emotional intelligence is an essential factor of life success, perhaps even more so than IQ. Emotional intelligence is the ability to understand your own (**intrapersonal**) and others' (**interpersonal**) emotions. These skills are important for a variety of reasons. Understanding your own emotions and those of others and being able to regulate and respond appropriately are keys to lifelong success. In his book *Outliers: The Story of Success*, Malcolm Gladwell (2008) tells the story of a young man with an IQ and technology savvy similar to Bill Gates's, yet he is not nearly as successful. Gladwell discusses how this man's social-emotional skills, or lack of them, contribute to his inability to achieve success. One of his biggest obstacles, according to Gladwell, is his perception that the world is out to get him; his issues seem to stem from a lack of emotional intelligence. He doesn't respond with appropriate emotion to many situations. He doesn't correctly interpret the emotions and actions of others. Early childhood educators can help children develop these competencies so they can understand the world they grow into and excel rather than be limited like the man Gladwell describes.

In her article "Social and Emotional Learning: What Is It? How Can We Use It to Help Our Children?" Robin Stern, PhD (2012), cites Dr. James Comer, a national leader in social and emotional learning, who told a group at Columbia Teachers College at a November 1999 conference about the impact school and home settings can have on children's development. Comer reported that settings that support social and emotional learning and competence can make a huge difference in children's lives. The difference, Comer claims, is equal to the difference in the outcome between throwing seeds on cement versus planting them in enriched soil. This excellent analogy highlights the significance of social-emotional development.

This section will address:

- Emotional recognition, expression, and regulation: Recognizing, expressing, and regulating emotions are important life skills. Teachers have many opportunities to introduce, teach, and enhance these developing skills.

- Managing difficult emotions: It's a fact of life: young children cope with difficult emotions. Fortunately, there are many strategies for responding to and helping children manage difficult emotions that also teach children coping and behavior skills.

Emotional Recognition, Expression, and Regulation

Children are born with little ability to control themselves physically or emotionally. Much of their early development involves gaining control and learning to self-regulate. Children progress from not being able to control much movement to rolling over, sitting up, crawling, standing, and walking. This same progression occurs when they attempt to control their emotions. While this development is less obvious, it is just as important. They move from crying to meeting most of their own needs, from temper tantrums to saying, "I mad," from waiting their turn for a desired toy to laughing with a friend over a shared experience. While they do so, they are demonstrating growth in three key **emotional intelligence** competencies: recognizing, expressing, and regulating emotions. People who cannot control or express their emotions experience less success socially; they have fewer personal and professional achievements and satisfactions. You hold out your hands to children attempting to take their first steps. You should also guide children who are attempting to understand and manage their complex emotions.

Teachers play an essential role in emotional development. Emotions affect young infants from their earliest stages. Your emotions serve as models and sources of feedback for infants as they begin to develop and grow. Research shows that the amount and nature of the emotional interactions young children engage in affect their development. Joseph and Strain have found that "when educators teach children the key skills they need to understand their emotions and the emotions of others, handle conflicts, problem solve, and develop relationships with peers, their problem behavior decreases and their social skills improve" (as quoted in Fox and Lentini 2006, 2). Your interactions and modeling are essential strategies for fostering this critical emotional development.

Culture and family dynamics play significant roles in emotional recognition and expression. Many family rules for emotional expression and spoken and unspoken cultural norms exist. Understanding children's family and cultural contexts helps you support children's individual development.

RECOGNIZING EMOTIONS

Goal: Children can recognize their own emotions in developmentally appropriate ways.

❑ Teachers create opportunities for children to name their own and others' emotions.

❑ When children are expressing an emotion, teachers help them identify and name it.

❑ Teachers **scaffold** children's understanding of emotions.

❑ Teachers discuss emotions and feelings throughout the day.

❑ Teachers plan specific activities, such as role play or matching games, to support emotional recognition.

❑ Children are given opportunities to predict or reflect others' emotions in stories, play situations, or role plays.

EXPRESSING EMOTIONS

Goal: Children can express their emotions appropriately.

❑ Teachers acknowledge and respond to children's expressed emotions.

❑ Teachers help children name their expressed emotions.

❑ Teachers help children build vocabularies to help them express their emotions.

❑ Teachers allow children to express positive and negative emotions.

❑ Teachers validate children's emotions.

Did you know? Acknowledge, respond to, and validate children's emotions. None of these actions has to indicate agreement with the emotion or the way children choose to express their feelings. When you acknowledge children's emotions, you demonstrate respect. This helps children stop focusing on expressing their emotions, directs their energies toward regulating their feelings, and helps them get their needs met. Not acknowledging their emotions has the opposite effect. For example, ignoring infants' cries only makes them feel less secure and more anxious. They cry more. When you respond to cries, infants don't receive the message, "You were right to cry." Instead, they understand, "I heard you crying, and I am here for you."

❑ Children are not punished or shamed for expressing emotions.

❑ Teachers model and teach emotional expression.

❑ Teachers have the same expectations and responses to boys' and girls' emotional expressions.

Did you know? It's easy to fall back on stereotypes when it comes to emotional expression. Telling a boy who is crying to toughen up, and giving a girl in the same situation a hug are perfect examples. While **temperament** and gender differences certainly play roles in children's emotional expressions, teachers should not reinforce stereotypes. Give both genders equal opportunity and support to express their emotions.

❑ Children can express emotions throughout the day during activities such as art, play, group times, and dramatic play.

❑ When children are resolving conflicts, they are encouraged to reflect on and express emotions.

REGULATING EMOTIONS

Goal: Children are taught how to regulate their emotions appropriately.

❑ Teachers plan specific activities, such as role playing or matching games, to practice emotional regulation.

❑ Teachers model and teach appropriate emotional responses to daily incidents.

❑ Teachers respond to children and validate their feelings even when they don't agree with them.

❑ Teachers use stories to teach children about emotional regulation.

❑ Teachers provide opportunities for children to predict emotional responses to situations.

❑ Teachers teach children ways to think about their emotions and behaviors before reacting to a situation.

❑ Teachers discuss and teach about the perspectives of others.

❑ Teachers teach and model effective coping strategies.

❑ Teachers respect children's individual methods of emotional regulation.

❑ Learning materials and the environment are developmentally appropriate.

❑ Rules and expectations in the learning environment are explicit and developmentally appropriate.

Did you know? What do developmentally appropriate environments, materials, and expectations have to do with emotional regulation? If there aren't enough toys and materials, if the environment isn't warm and comfortable, if there are no soft, calming spaces, or if expectations are unrealistic or change a lot, children will grapple with difficult emotions regularly. Their emotions will be hard to regulate. This almost guarantees fighting, biting, and angry outbursts. A warm, inviting, peaceful community provides some external help for children while they work on regulating their emotions. It minimizes the difficult emotions they must cope with.

Managing Difficult Emotions

In their early years, young children are faced daily with brand-new experiences. Some of these are situations in which young children can't succeed on their own or are dependent on others to meet their needs. This tires and frustrates most adults. It's worse for young children, who can't understand or regulate their emotions yet. All young children experience strong negative emotions sometimes. You should see these moments as teaching and relationship-building opportunities. If children learn how to cope with these emotions while feeling supported and loved, they will learn to manage these emotions themselves more quickly. If they are shamed or punished for their feelings, they will continue struggling. You should understand these moments as opportunities to prepare and equip children with important skills for the future.

Note: Some children express difficult emotions more often or in more challenging ways. It is not always possible or a good idea for child care programs to manage extreme behaviors without support. Partner with family members and other community resources to help children whose emotions overwhelm them and their teachers.

MANAGING DIFFICULT EMOTIONS

Goal: Children develop the skills and abilities they need to manage difficult emotions successfully.

❑ Activities and equipment are set up to promote success and minimize frustration.

❑ When children indicate they are experiencing difficult emotions, teachers observe and record potential triggers, effective techniques and strategies, and types of reactions.

Did you know? When children are having prolonged or repeated challenges with their emotions and behaviors, keep a log or record to track their behavior and emotions. This can be very useful. Within a few days to a week or two, patterns begin to emerge. Maybe children are more reactive at certain times of day or after particular types of experiences. Making small tweaks to their daily experience can make a world of difference. A detailed record or log is also useful for conversations with family members or community resources.

❑ Teachers focus on the root cause, not the symptoms, of the difficult emotion.

❑ Teachers focus on the child's behavior, not the child herself, when responding to the child.

Did you know? Focusing on the child's behavior, rather than on the child herself, is an important concept for teachers to understand and apply. It's the difference between saying, "You're a bad kid!" and saying, "Your behavior was bad, but you are a good kid," when unwanted behavior occurs. If a child feels hurt or ashamed, thinking about and learning how to change an unwanted behavior will be difficult, and the unwanted behavior will likely occur again. Teachers should always use behavior-based statements such as, "Hanna, when you took Alaysia's doll, it made her feel sad," rather than using blaming or child-focused statements like, "Hanna, stop being naughty." Not only does a focus on behaviors work to eliminate unwanted behaviors, but it also models effective communication strategies for the child—a bonus.

❑ Teachers realize that many behaviors are expressions of fear, stress, anxiety, worry, or lack of self-worth. They respond accordingly.

❑ Children are taught appropriate ways to express, rather than suppress, their emotions.

❑ Teachers collaborate with family members and/or professionals when children consistently express difficult emotions.

Section 11

Positive Behavior Guidance

Children's behavior is often challenging. That doesn't mean children themselves are *bad* or *naughty*. They are simply experimenting with getting their needs met and interacting with the world. Challenging behavior often results from emotions that children don't know how to cope with or regulate. They are trying to learn about or manipulate their world. Challenging behavior always happens for a reason. Educators must find out why it is occurring and use these moments as teaching opportunities. How you respond to children in these moments can have a significant impact on their lives (Jacobson 2008).

Early childhood educators request guidance on behavior more than on any other topic. Providers are often looking for ways to stop challenging behaviors. But that is unrealistic. Children are only starting to learn the skills they need to manage their behaviors. Their ability to understand and regulate their emotions is just emerging. Their capacity for controlling their responses is limited. Their curiosity about the world is limitless (and should not be reined in). You need to recognize the connection between children's emotional and social competencies and their behavior. When you do, you can see behavior challenges as teaching opportunities and as forms of communication. You can minimize challenging behaviors, ease your own frustration, and help children develop positive social skills.

Suitable spaces and teaching approaches help prevent and manage behavioral challenges. Prevention is key, but it is impossible to avoid all behavior challenges when working with young children. Building strong social and emotional skills and abilities in children lessens behavioral challenges. How you respond to behaviors is equally important. Teachers' responses commonly range from the belief that children should be punished to ignoring or indulging their demands. You should respond in ways that promote development and teach the child. **Behavior guidance** is the best approach. *Guidance* is the key word; guidance should be the intent behind all of your responses. You should never punish, shame, or condemn the behavior or the child. **Punishment** doesn't work and certainly has no place in a program focused on learning and development. Your goal is to guide children's behavior so they can learn to get their needs met appropriately. Each child is an individual, so different approaches and strategies are needed for the children in your care. When children are taught effective social-emotional skills and strategies, only about 4 percent of behavioral challenges remain (Fox and Lentini 2006). Of course, some behavioral issues are indicators of larger problems. You should treat such behaviors as symptoms and work collaboratively with families and other professionals to support the child.

This section will address:

- A positive approach to guiding behavior: strategies to use behavior challenges as teaching opportunities and to guide children's behavior in positive ways

A Positive Approach to Guiding Behavior

Guiding children's behavior is an awesome responsibility, yet many adults do not plan for or think about it. You should consider the moments when children are struggling with their behavior as ideal moments to guide them. Children look to adults for help when they don't have the knowledge, skills, or abilities to go in the right direction. If adults punish or ignore their unspoken need for direction, children stay lost and may choose unhealthy or challenging paths on their own. You can guide behavior by setting up the environment, teaching and practicing skills with them, and responding appropriately to their conflicts or behavioral challenges.

UNACCEPTABLE FORMS OF PUNISHMENT

Goal: We do not tolerate any forms of abuse, verbal or physical, in our program.

❑ Children are never teased, belittled, called names, or otherwise verbally abused.

❑ No biases are tolerated toward children because of their or their families' diversity or ability, including a child's own stage of development.

❑ Teachers protect children from physical and verbal harm.

BEHAVIOR GUIDANCE APPROACH

Goal: We provide an approach to behavior guidance that treats children's challenging behaviors as opportunities to teach and support rather than punish or condemn.

❑ Teachers' responses to behavior are considered teaching strategies and used as such.

❑ Teachers recognize that developing strong and trusting relationships deters challenging behaviors.

❑ Challenging behaviors are seen as opportunities to support children's development.

❑ Teachers are knowledgeable about developmentally appropriate behaviors, needs, and abilities. Their expectations of children's behavior reflect this knowledge.

❑ Responses to challenging behavior are individualized.

❑ Teachers use calm voices and demeanor when responding to children's challenging behavior.

❑ Consequences to challenging behavior are natural and logical.

❑ Time-outs and isolation are not used to respond to challenging behavior. Children can take a break from an activity and engage briefly in a calming activity if needed.

❑ The behavior, not the child, is the focus of all behavior guidance.

PREVENTIVE ENVIRONMENTAL STRATEGIES

Goal: Our program environment minimizes or prevents challenging behaviors and emotions.

❑ Children are not exposed to violence in the program, including through media, images, books, materials, or adult conversations.

❑ Materials and activities complement the cognitive abilities of children to avoid frustration.

❑ The program environment includes spaces that are warm, cozy, and comforting.

❑ The program environment includes spaces that allow children to safely be alone or in small groups of peers.

❑ The learning environment includes space and/or materials designated for working out frustration or resolving problems.

❑ Enough materials are available so children do not always have to share or wait for a turn.

❑ The program environment is organized to promote independence and mastery.

❑ The program environment is organized to reflect behavioral expectations. For example, it has no long hallways if children are expected not to run inside.

PREVENTIVE TEACHING STRATEGIES

Goal: We use teaching strategies that minimize or prevent challenging behaviors and emotions.

❑ Children are not required or forced to participate in activities or experiences.

❑ Activities and materials are challenging yet achievable.

❑ Teachers teach problem solving and provide many opportunities to practice.

❑ Teachers teach conflict-resolution skills and provide many opportunities to practice.

❑ Teachers teach children how to consider another's perspective and discuss perspective in many situations.

❑ "Rules" or expectations are clear, positively stated, and often reviewed and support independence and mastery.

Did you know? Posting a list of rules on the wall is a start, but children are unlikely to understand, remember, or know how to meet them. Instead, develop expectations with the children. State expectations positively by describing what children can do rather than what they can't do. Discuss and practice the expectations regularly. Acknowledging a child's compliance can go a long way: "Wow, Kota. I see you are finished with the magnets, and you are putting them away before you choose another activity. I appreciate that you remembered to do that."

❑ Teachers help children understand the differences between *tattling* and *telling*.

❑ Behavioral expectations are aligned with developmental abilities.

Did you know? It's important that your expectations for behavior are realistic. For example, if you expect young toddlers to share, you are all but asking for behavioral challenges to occur. If a certain expectation, material, or activity seems to cause behavioral challenges, it's probably not developmentally appropriate.

❑ Experiences and activities are inclusive of a wide range of interests and abilities.

❑ Children are not expected to share or work together at all times.

❑ Children are never labeled by their behavior; for example, they are not called *bossy, bully, naughty,* or *mean.*

❑ Children have many choices available at all times, including group time.

❑ Children's natural tendencies to play physically and to engage in active imaginative play are allowed.

Did you know? If you have worked in an early childhood classroom, you have met a superhero once or twice or seen a toy turned into a weapon a time or two. This type of imaginative, active play is troubling to many teachers, but it is developmentally appropriate. Simply saying no to this imaginative play does little to minimize it. You can, however, create boundaries so children remain safe and respectful while exploring their curiosity and imaginations.

❑ Routines and schedules are consistent yet flexible.

❑ All teachers in the space have the same expectations and routines of behavior.

IN-THE-MOMENT STRATEGIES

Goal: We use teaching strategies that help children diffuse and solve challenges as they occur.

❑ Teachers use their knowledge of developmentally appropriate expectations and behaviors to guide their response to children's behaviors.

❑ Teachers encourage and support children's attempts to solve their own problems or challenges.

❑ Teachers model problem solving, communicating, and listening skills while resolving conflicts or responding to behavior.

❑ Teachers acknowledge the needs, emotions, and perspectives of all involved.

❑ Teachers refer to previous learning to remind children of expectations.

❑ Teachers do not ignore harmful physical or verbal behaviors even if the children resolve their own conflicts.

❑ Teachers say "No" only when necessary. "No" is accompanied by an explanation.

❑ Teachers document challenging behaviors to understand patterns and underlying causes (following confidentiality regulations).

❑ Teachers express unconditional kindness to children who express negative behavior.

❑ If a child has damaged a social relationship (for example, had a tantrum in front of the group or pulled a friend's hair), the teacher helps the child regain entry into social play after the incident.

❑ Children are not required to say "Sorry" unless they feel and understand remorse.

Did you know? Telling children to say "Sorry" is well intentioned but yields little result. Children learn that saying it amounts to a get-out-of-jail-free pass. What you really want is for children to feel sorry. This takes more effort. Asking them to care for the peer they harmed, to repair the toy or material they damaged, or to cheer up the friend whose feelings they have hurt is more likely to help them truly feel sorry than just saying it.

SUPPORT FOR EXTREME BEHAVIORS AND/OR EMOTIONS

Goal: We support children while they learn to cope with and regulate occasional extreme emotions or behaviors.

❑ Teachers recognize that extreme behaviors are indicators of other challenges and work toward understanding their cause.

❑ Teachers have soothing toys and materials in the environment to manage anger, anxiety, and stress.

❑ When children have repeated or severe challenging behaviors, teachers work with families and other professionals to support them and meet their needs.

❑ Our program has an established protocol for responding to repeated or severe challenging behaviors. Families have been made aware of and agreed to our protocol when they enrolled.

❑ Teachers do not hold grudges, and they start each day with a clean slate.

❑ Teachers show interest, caring, and kindness to all children equally.

Section 12

Approaches to Learning

In the past few years, **approaches to learning** (ATL), or learning dispositions, have been added to the list of developmental domains that educators should focus on. Approaches to learning include the ways children and adults feel about learning, prepare to learn, and participate in learning. They focus on *how* children learn versus *what* they learn. Approaches to learning are a blend of cognitive and social-emotional skills and abilities that allow children to learn, including self-regulation, **delayed gratification**, perseverance, curiosity, focus, self-control, and engagement. They are included in part 3 because their development is interdependent with social and emotional development. Children who lack healthy social and emotional skills won't approach learning positively and vice versa. Consider learning how to read as an example of the way learning approaches work. Children must be motivated and engaged to keep looking at books and listening to read-aloud stories. They need to be curious about symbols or letters on the page. They must persist despite setbacks like mispronunciations and irregular words. They must try various strategies to link letters and sounds together and make meaning. These qualities are approaches to learning, or learning dispositions. Without them, children have a much harder time learning to read. When they lack well-developed approaches to learning, they face many challenges in trying to learn and develop. Their negative experiences can snowball and eventually lead them to disengage from formal learning experiences altogether.

The Collaborative for Academic, Social, and Emotional Learning (CASEL) sums up the vital importance of both learning approaches and social-emotional competence:

> To succeed in school, students need to be engaged, interested, and excited to be there. They need to know how to focus their attention on their work, keep trying even when they get discouraged or face setbacks, work effectively with other students and adults, and be good communicators and problem-solvers. These skills form a foundation for young people's success not just in school, but in their adult lives as members of the community, as productive workers, and as parents. (2007, 1)

Well-developed learning approaches positively influence learners' **resilience**. Well-developed learning skills are like keys. No matter how smart learners are or how high their IQ, if they don't have the right keys, they can't open many doors.

This section will address:

- Self-skills: Methods to positively support skills that relate to the self: self-esteem, self-concept, self-regulation, and self-confidence.

- Approaches to learning skills: Teaching practices that nurture approaches to learning, or skills that help a child (or adult) learn, such as curiosity and perseverance.

Self-Skills

Developing a sense of self is one of the earliest, most ongoing tasks in children's lives. Infants begin by discovering their toes and fingers. Slowly they realize they are separate beings with their own desires and abilities. Soon they begin to notice the world around them. They start shaping their perception of who they are and how they fit into the world. Children see themselves first in simple terms. They are their mother's child, their sister's sibling. Maybe they have black hair and brown eyes. Then they begin attributing characteristics and traits to themselves: "I am nice," or "I am good at art." Children develop their perceptions using feedback they receive from the adults, peers, environment, and experiences they encounter each day. When their efforts are received with encouragement and joy, they internalize those responses. When they are punished often or labeled, they begin to identify with those experiences. How the adults in children's worlds behave, even when not specifically interacting with children, can influence their sense of self as well. When children see the adults in their lives helping others, they begin to identify with that behavior and often mimic it. If they see adults in their lives being dishonest, they learn to behave that way.

Self-regulation is an equally important concept. In fact, it is so important, it is highlighted in the landmark book *From Neurons to Neighborhoods*: "The growth of self-regulation is a cornerstone of early childhood development that cuts across all domains of behavior" (National Research Council and Institute of Medicine 2000). Self-regulation skills help people respond and react to achieve the best possible outcomes for themselves. They are like internal yield and stop signs.

Helping children to develop sense of self and self-regulation is not difficult, but it should be done intentionally. These skills help children have strong, positive images of themselves, their abilities, and what they can accomplish. Strong and positive self-skills are immeasurably valuable to their overall health and well-being.

SELF-CONCEPT AND SELF-ESTEEM

Goal: All children receive support in developing positive self-concept and self-esteem.

❑ Each child is individually welcomed each day.

❑ Teachers use children's names instead of nicknames.

❑ Photos of children and their families are visible.

❑ Teachers recognize and embrace the diversity of the children and families in the program.

❑ Teachers respect children's individual preferences and choices.

❑ Teachers plan opportunities for children to get to know and think about themselves, such as creating self-portraits, writing books about their families, or sharing items from home.

❑ Teachers acknowledge specific traits, characteristics, and accomplishments of each child.

❑ Children are never compared to one another regarding abilities or behaviors.

❑ Teachers encourage rather than praise children.

Did you know? The distinction between encouragement and praise is important. Encouragement is meant to inspire perseverance. Praise expresses approval or admiration. When children are growing and learning rapidly, your encouragement can give them the gentle nudge they need to keep trying. When you overpraise children—for example, automatically saying, "Good job"—you send the message that completing something is the goal, when hard work and progress should be the goals. Too much praise for achievements can actually cause children to shy away from trying new things; they become afraid to fail, to not be worthy of the praise they are used to receiving. Consistently responding with genuine encouragement takes practice and focus to master, but it is an excellent way for teachers to support a child's self-esteem and self-concept.

❑ Teachers focus primarily on efforts, not outcomes.

Did you know? Everyone has heard about parents who give children money for every A on their report cards or about the children on a sports team who receive trophies even when they're in last place. The intentions were good, but the rewards do not lead to ongoing or long-term results. Children start to perform only for the material reward, which is **extrinsic motivation**. Your goal is to support children's **internal motivation**. They need to want to do well, keep improving, and try harder. Focusing on children's progress is more important than their end results. It's easy to focus on progress when children are still infants. Consider them learning to roll over. You clap and cheer at every millimeter they can move. You wouldn't consider responding to or encouraging them only if they roll over all the way. Remember to keep your focus on gradual progress and on effort as children grow and mature.

❑ Teachers ask children about their interests and experiences and demonstrate sustained interest by following up on previous conversations.

❑ Teachers recognize children's emerging self-awareness when they use words like *me* and *mine*.

SELF-REGULATION

Goal: Opportunities are provided for children to develop self-regulation skills.

❑ Teachers provide predictability in the environment and daily routines.

❑ Teachers promote awareness and acceptance of personal feelings.

❑ Teachers understand and maintain developmentally appropriate expectations for children in their care.

❑ Teachers help children develop their ability to focus and pay attention.

❑ Teachers do not expect children to pay attention for inappropriate lengths of time.

❑ Teachers give children appropriate choices and options throughout the day.

❑ Teachers help children identify available and preferable choices.

❑ Children's preferences and decisions are respected and supported, if they are safe.

❑ Teachers model self-regulation.

❑ Children are given opportunities to delay gratification regularly.

Did you know? Have you ever wanted something badly but had to wait? How did it feel? Were you able to do it? Children experience this feeling regularly. Learning to delay gratification or wait for what you want is a difficult but essential life skill. Think of the medical students who attend four years of medical school and work long hours for low pay for years to become doctors. They need the ability to delay gratification and endure the challenges of those many years to realize their dreams. You can help children learn to delay gratification throughout the day. For example, you can monitor how many children can play in a certain area and ask children to wait their turn when it is full. When children interrupt you while you're talking, you can gently signal them to wait.

❑ Teachers assist children in solving problems and help them weigh the pros and cons of various actions.

❑ Children are given the opportunity to reflect on previous decisions and experiences.

❑ Children play age- and ability-appropriate games that require and reinforce self-regulation.

❑ Teachers do not unnecessarily interrupt children when they are speaking or playing.

SELF-CONFIDENCE

Goal: Children receive the support they need to develop self-confidence.

❑ Children receive more acknowledgment for their progress and efforts than for their results.

❑ Children are encouraged to feel pride in themselves, their abilities, their decisions, and other accomplishments.

❑ Teachers **scaffold** skills and expectations so children don't become frustrated.

❑ Teachers acknowledge progress.

Did you know? Consider how adults react to an infant's attempts to walk. We respond with glee as they try to stand up, clap enthusiastically when they begin cruising around the room holding on to furniture, and eagerly encourage their first steps. We don't hold back our enthusiasm until they master walking, and we certainly don't get upset with them when their first steps result in tumbles. Yet, as children get older we often forget to praise their efforts and progress and instead focus on achievements and success. Focusing on effort and progress will not only result in more success, it will also motivate children to confidently try more things, even if they won't initially succeed.

❑ Teachers plan experiences that allow children to succeed.

❑ Teachers plan experiences that challenge children.

❑ The rules of the program are clear and consistent, so children understand its boundaries and expectations.

❑ Children have lots of opportunities to practice emerging skills.

❑ Children are never tested or put on the spot to demonstrate or perform a skill.

❑ Children's physical attributes are never judged or compared to those of others.

❑ Teachers help children establish and work toward personal goals.

Approaches to Learning Skills

"When a baby experiences a secure attachment and feels safe and protected, she develops the confidence that allows her to explore, try new things, and make mistakes. This confidence and willingness to experiment is what leads to competence as a young child and later as an adult" (Mooney 2010, 121). As children get to know themselves in their early years, as they develop confidence and willingness to experiment, they also begin to develop approaches to life and learning. These approaches are a collection of skills, perspectives, and attitudes that children use unconsciously and that influence all of their experiences. Well-developed **approaches to learning skills** support children's school success. For example, researchers have found direct correlations between approaches to learning skills and school achievement. Researcher Walter Mischel and his associates found a correlation between four-year-olds who could delay gratification and future performance in academic and social situations (Mischel, Shoda, and Rodriguez 1989).

Strong approaches to learning skills also help develop resiliency. Resiliency is a critical life skill that can protect children from the effects of adversity and life challenges. Resilient children still face struggles. But they are better able to cope with and manage struggles. Caring adults contribute to children's resiliency.

INITIATIVE AND CURIOSITY

Goal: Children's curiosity and initiative are nurtured.

- ❑ The learning environment is organized with ample and varied materials.

- ❑ Discovery is a primary goal of many activities and experiences.

- ❑ Few materials, toys, or books (if any) in the learning environment are based on commercial characters.

- ❑ Materials and activities are primarily open-ended and nurture creativity.

- ❑ Materials and activities reflect society's diversity.

- ❑ Children are encouraged to ask questions and express interests.

- ❑ Children are encouraged to predict what will happen next or in the future.

- ❑ Cause and effect are discussed and explored.

- ❑ Simple and complex choices are offered to children regularly.

- ❑ Children's experiences are varied. Materials are rotated occasionally.

- ❑ Art experiences are process oriented rather than product oriented.

Did you know? Process-oriented art is about experience, textures, tools, and the creative process. Product-oriented art is about the end result. Product art is often referred to as *crafts*. If you have a specific product in mind, a model for children to copy, or a right or wrong way of doing an art task, it is product oriented. While crafts can teach some skills, like following directions or cutting, they do not nurture creativity or promote flexible thinking or curiosity. Crafts can also send negative messages if a child isn't able to copy the model or color inside the lines on a coloring page. Avoid lines to color outside of in early art experiences; provide only wide-open spaces for children to create masterpieces.

❑ Outdoor time offers children an opportunity to explore their natural environment.

❑ Children regularly engage in scientific learning.

❑ When children are struggling with a new skill or task, teachers do not intervene or do it for them; teachers can scaffold the task or assist the child if necessary.

Did you know? Building children's "I can do it!" attitude is worthwhile. Learning new skills takes patience and practice, so allow children to have those experiences. The next time they face a challenge, they will believe they can overcome it. When children ask for help or become frustrated, respond by supporting their attempts or modeling the task rather than doing it for them. Keep in mind that the end goal is building children's initiative and belief in their own abilities.

❑ Most materials and activities in the environment can be used without teachers' support.

PERSEVERANCE, ENGAGEMENT, AND MOTIVATION

Goal: We develop and practice children's perseverance, engagement, and motivation.

❑ Teachers do not attempt to motivate children by offering external rewards.

❑ Children can participate in long-term, ongoing projects.

❑ Children's work is not interrupted or stopped unnecessarily.

❑ Teachers extend children's experiences and learning.

❑ The environment reflects children's work.

❑ Teachers use children's interests to plan and implement activities.

❑ Children are encouraged to keep trying if they have not succeeded in their first attempts.

❑ Teachers get to know children and understand their unique goals and motivation.

PROBLEM SOLVING AND CRITICAL THINKING

Goal: We encourage children to think critically and problem solve.

❏ Adults do not interfere when children work together to solve a problem.

❏ Children are encouraged to plan and direct their own work and processes.

❏ Teachers help children develop and practice the skills needed to solve problems; this can occur during actual conflicts or when no problem exists.

❏ Teachers intervene in children's problem solving only when necessary.

❏ Teachers model problem solving.

❏ Teachers help children reason.

❏ Teachers ask children open-ended questions and make open-ended comments.

❏ Teachers often ask *why*, *how*, and *what if* questions.

❏ Children are encouraged to consider the outcomes of varied situations or decisions.

❏ Teachers use strategies like "Plan, Do, Review" or "What do we know? What do we want to learn? and What have we learned? (KWL)." These help children think about experiences before, during, and after they occur.

❏ Teachers ask children what they think.

❏ Teachers encourage and nurture creative thinking and ideas even when they are not plausible or correct.

❏ Teachers plan activities that allow experimenting.

❏ Materials in the environment encourage exploring.

❏ Teachers limit the number of activities that emphasize right-or-wrong answers or methods.

Section 13

Family Support and Involvement

Support for families is essential. Parenting is difficult, and a support network helps all families. All families can benefit from being part of a community. They can thrive within a supportive network. When child care providers and families work collaboratively and support one another, children benefit.

Parents and other adults tasked with daily care of children are sometimes confronted by life challenges. These may include teen pregnancy, poverty, lack of food or shelter, divorce, job loss, extreme stress, abuse, lack of education, and language challenges. Life challenges can prevent adults from parenting effectively. To compound the difficulties, adults who did not form strong attachments or social and emotional skills as children will be challenged when they try to model and provide those for their own children. Teachers cannot meet all of a family's needs. But you should consider yourself part of each family's community and support network. Families need resilience to face typical and sometimes extreme life challenges. They can develop or strengthen their resiliency within a network of positive relationships and support. In fact, secure family connections are the single most critical factor in reducing negative outcomes for children (Sesame Street Resilience Initiative 2011).

Because families interact with you regularly, they often develop trusting relationships with you. Recognize the value of this trust and the relationship they have with you. Help families lessen or eliminate barriers that prevent them from supporting their children. According to the Center for Social Policy, "They [families] are much more likely to accept assistance and advice from someone they have chosen themselves, whom they see every day, than to accept services offered only after problems emerge or they are identified as 'at risk'" (CSSP 2007, 1–2). This is true of all families regardless of education, socioeconomic status, and life challenges. A "we're in this together" mentality and a partnership should be the goal of your relationships with families. This means you need to understand each family's culture, perspective on child rearing, and parenting goals. Programs for families should provide education, resources, and support to build up current parenting abilities. Families should be told about program policies, approaches, and philosophies so they can work with them, rather than at odds with them. Aligned messages, shared support, and a strength-building approach provide children positive foundations on which to grow and thrive.

This section will address:

- Family connections: Being connected with other families is an important way to prevent family stress and trauma and increase family wellness. Child care programs can easily support and facilitate many opportunities for families to connect.

- Family resources and support: By sharing resources or providing information about community resources, a program can support the emotional health of children even when they're not attending the program.

- Program resources: There are multiple ways to support the development of social-emotional skills in young children each day. Providing teachers with expert resources and teaching materials increases their ability to teach effectively.

Family Connections

Deep, meaningful partnerships with families are important to healthy child care experiences. Family members and teachers need to support one another and work toward the same goals for the child. Many parents may not expect or are wary of such relationships. For this reason, teachers are responsible for developing positive relationships with families just as they are for building positive relationships with children. Be mindful and respectful of families' values and cultural beliefs. In positive relationships, people do not impose their beliefs and values on one another. Your relationship with families should be professional, warm, supportive, and respectful.

CONNECTIONS BETWEEN PARENTS/FAMILIES

Goal: All families have positive relationships with other families. No family is isolated or lacks support.

❑ New families are introduced to families in the program. They are encouraged to develop relationships.

❑ Mentor families are appointed for new families.

❑ A comfortable and welcoming space exists for families to gather and meet.

❑ Networking opportunities, such as Tuesday morning coffee or quarterly family nights, are offered regularly.

❑ A place exists for families to share information or make requests, such as a bulletin board and/or parent group.

❑ Shared services, such as carpooling and babysitters, are encouraged.

❑ Family events are planned at different times so all families can attend.

❑ Family members besides parents are encouraged to participate in the program.

❑ Volunteer opportunities are offered to parents, both in and out of the program.

❑ Diversity is embraced, respected, and considered in planning family events and opportunities.

CONNECTIONS BETWEEN PARENTS/FAMILIES AND TEACHERS

Goal: All families are connected to the program. No family is isolated or lacks support.

❑ Time is set aside daily for teachers to connect with parents of infants and other nonverbal children.

❑ Time is set aside weekly for teachers to connect with parents of verbal children.

❑ Teachers treat the arrival of a new child as the beginning of a collaborative relationship.

❑ Discussions with families are supportive and respectful.

❑ All teachers respect the parents' role as a child's primary source of care and first teacher.

❑ Communication between families and teachers occurs regularly. It can be by phone, e-mail, and notes. It is always confidential.

❑ Teachers' advice is based on developmentally appropriate practice, not personal experience.

❑ The program has an open-door policy. Parents can observe their children.

❑ Conferences are used to build strong relationships and educate parents about their child's development. Conferences also report academic achievements.

❑ Mothers, fathers, and other guardians are equally included in the program.

❑ Parents know that teachers are mandated reporters.

❑ Teachers ask and learn about each individual family, including cultural preferences, traditions, parenting styles, and goals for children.

❑ Teachers take parents' requests and concerns seriously. They respond respectfully in a timely manner.

❑ Relationships between teachers and parents are professional.

Bonus Checklist

❏ Teachers conduct home visits annually or more often. They discuss early childhood development, the child's progress and development, and opportunities for partnership between the program and family. This is also the time to answer the families' questions and build relationships with them.

Family Resources and Support

Families are bombarded with information about parenting from many sources. Even the savviest parent has a hard time weeding through the variety of perspectives, advice, and theories to find meaningful information. Families are also under more stress than ever before. They often lack extended family nearby to lend support. When they are coping with multiple challenges, parents often don't feel successful *as* parents. You can serve as a reliable and trusted resource for them. You can help parents identify credible and relevant information. You can also become a trusted and comforting mentor as they navigate the wonderful, yet challenging, responsibilities of parenting.

Learn to appreciate the influence and the amount of trust families often put in your advice and opinions. Sort through your biases and preferences to make sure the support and resources you offer families meet their needs and are based on best practices.

FAMILY EDUCATION AND RESOURCES

Goal: Families use teachers as reliable and dependable sources of information and education to help them parent successfully.

❏ Parenting education, within the program or from an outside source, is offered on topics that include the following:
   ❏ child development
   ❏ parenting strategies
   ❏ work/life balance
   ❏ communication
   ❏ stress reduction
   ❏ developmentally appropriate practice (DAP) and program curriculum
   ❏ positive child guidance
   ❏ social and emotional development
   ❏ social and emotional skills (for parents or other adults)

❑ The program lowers barriers to effective relationships, such as language.

❑ Families are informed of the program's collaborative approach from the beginning.

❑ An up-to-date lending and resource library is available to families.

❑ Resources on health issues are always readily available, including materials relevant to the families in your program, such as the following:
   ❑ **sudden infant death syndrome (SIDS)**
   ❑ **shaken baby syndrome**
   ❑ food shelves
   ❑ crisis services, such as crisis nurseries and abuse hotlines
   ❑ community health services
   ❑ parenting classes or groups

❑ The program offers a list of referrals, and families are aware they are available.

Program Resources

Families see child care programs and teachers as trusted and reliable resources on child development. If they want to learn more, they often look to their children's teacher first. It's unlikely you will know every fact about every topic. But if you know of current, reliable, and relevant resources, you and the families can learn what you need to know.

PROGRAM RESOURCES

Goal: Our program has accurate and relevant resources about social-emotional development, resilience, and approaches to learning. These are available to families and teachers.

❑ Books, DVDs, and other relevant resources are available in our family lending library.

❑ Books, DVDs, and other relevant resources are available in our teachers' resource library.

❑ The program provides resources so teachers can support social-emotional development in their daily activities and lesson plans.

❑ The program provides resources so teachers can support the development of learning approaches in their daily activities and lesson plans.

❑ The program makes relevant children's books available to children and their families.

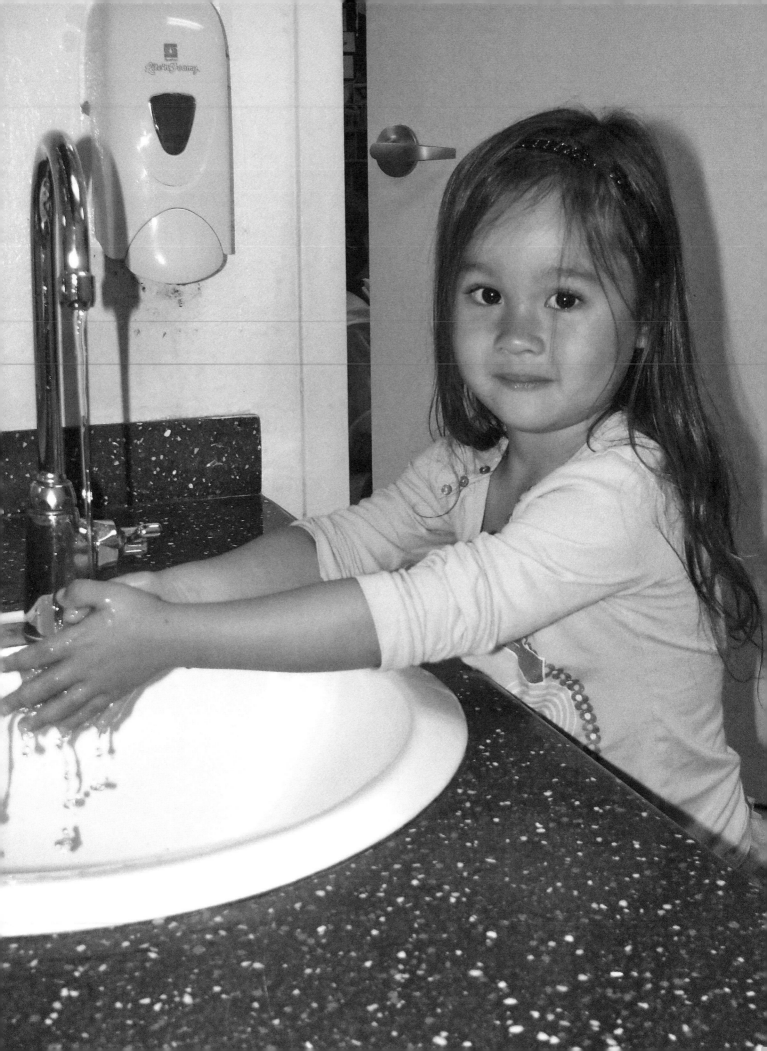

Part 4

Physical Health

Early childhood programs typically focus on children's physical, intellectual, social, and emotional development. To develop to their fullest, children must be healthy and ready to participate in the program. One of your primary goals is to protect the health of the children in your care. Most children arrive each day healthy and ready to learn and participate. Naturally, you want them to stay healthy. You can protect their health by **cleaning** toys, furniture, and spaces used by children, attending to hygiene, and caring for and maintaining the environment. Your own health will benefit from learning how to protect children.

For children to grow and develop, their physical needs must be met. Children need to be protected from the risks of illness and contaminants. Many of your daily practices help to protect you and the children from illness and other threats to their health. For example, you are probably already using hand washing to protect children's (and your own) health. You probably have a cleaning schedule to keep the environment neat and to minimize germs.

Even with these excellent hygiene practices in place, illness among children and adults is inevitable. To minimize outbreaks of illness or infection, you monitor children's health, exclude ill children, and possibly give medications required by a child's physician. Children's **allergies** and **chronic illnesses**, such as diabetes or **asthma**, also require routine attention from you and your program.

Besides preventing and minimizing the spread of illness, you protect children's health by carefully maintaining their daily environment. Hazards in the air and water affect all children and may have even greater impact on children with conditions like asthma.

Many resources are available to help you promote children's health. You are unlikely to have training as a medical or health professional, but sometimes you may feel as if you need it. You can do a lot to create and maintain a healthy program without being a doctor or a nurse! Most professionals working with children partner with health professionals to sort through available health information. Partnering is a very effective way to improve the overall health of your program. Your child care health consultant can help you identify goals for your program and sift through the technical information, which can sometimes seem overwhelming.

Throughout parts 4, 5, and 6 of *Healthy Children, Healthy Lives,* you will see references to *Caring for our Children: National Health and Safety Performance Standards.* This resource was developed by the American Academy of Pediatrics, the American Public Health Association, and the National Resource Center for Health and Safety in Child Care and Early Education with support from the U.S. Department of Health and Human Services (2011). This comprehensive resource is the basis for the regulations enacted by many states, the policies developed by many providers, and the criteria developed by many early childhood accreditation programs. It can enhance the quality in your early care and education program. These standards are considered the "gold standard" in promoting children's health in child care. We have used them throughout the checklists in this book. You can find the entire text of *Caring for Our Children* online at http://nrckids.org/.

Section 14

Health Promotion

Most children arrive at your early childhood program healthy and ready to explore. Each day, they have many opportunities to interact with you and the other children in the program. Every interaction brings special opportunities for learning and development of social and emotional skills. As an educator, you want children to interact freely and to have many chances to touch and explore, be messy, and use materials creatively alongside one another. One of the challenges associated with groups of children interacting together is the risk of illness, injury, or infection. A big part of your role is helping children remain healthy, learn good hygiene habits, and grow through their interactions with one another.

Young children are still learning the basic hygiene practices that protect them from illness and infection. They must rely on adults to model good practices and encourage them to learn and use good hygiene. They are just beginning to form the habits that will last a lifetime. So their early years are the perfect time for you to introduce health promotion skills and hygiene activities. You can promote good health by teaching such skills as hand washing and toothbrushing.

You need to know a great deal to plan a developmental program for young children. You also need to know a lot to support children's health and well-being. You should expect to rely on other important partners to promote the health of the children in your care. Partner with families and health professionals—and especially with a child care health consultant. Child care health consultants help programs establish healthy policies, train teachers in healthy practices, and stay up-to-date on emerging ideas and resources.

This section will address:

- Hand washing: Experts indicate that hand washing may be the most important health promotion activity undertaken in child care programs.

- Standard precautions: Providers can prevent the spread of **blood-borne pathogens** by practicing **standard precautions** in situations involving blood or body fluids contaminated by blood.

- Health information: Collecting and updating a wide variety of information helps programs to fully understand and promote children's health.

- Immunizations: A wide variety of vaccine-preventable illness can be addressed by using the recommended schedule for childhood **immunizations**.

- Dental/oral health: Toothbrushing and other oral and dental health practices prevent **cavities** and establish lifelong habits.

- Health consultation: Child care health consultants are invaluable supports to the work of child care professionals and programs.

Hand Washing

When working with young children, you will find yourself washing your hands many times a day. In fact, hand washing is so frequent that it easily becomes routine and loses its importance. You must resist becoming complacent about hand washing. It is of critical importance to your health and the health of the children you are caring for.

Hand washing is the best deterrent against illness, infection, and a wide range of illnesses. Children and adults who practice frequent and thorough hand washing are healthier (AAP, APHA, and NRC 2011). Hand washing is a simple, low-cost approach to stemming illness and infection, but it requires thoughtful training, adequate supplies, and regular reminders to be effective.

Young children are learning about hand washing. Although most of them enjoy interacting with water, their hand washing may be inconsistent and less thorough than it needs to be. Adults can model hand-washing procedures, encourage hand washing, and monitor children's hand washing. Learn about the importance of hand washing and incorporate it into children's healthy habits—doing so helps children throughout their lives. Besides the practices in the following checklists, consider creating two posters for each hand washing area in your program. First, post the times when hand washing is expected. Second, post a visual description of the hand-washing procedure. Whenever possible, use photographs so children who don't read yet can follow the steps independently. You can find examples of hand-washing posters on the National Resource Center for Health and Safety in Child Care and Early Education website (http://nrckids.org/).

STAFF MEMBERS AND VOLUNTEERS

Goal: Our program practices routine hand washing to ensure that we do not transmit illness and infection.

❑ Supplies for frequent and thorough hand washing are readily available. These include running water no colder than 60 degrees Fahrenheit and no hotter than 120 degrees Fahrenheit, liquid soap, and single-use towels or air dryers.

❑ Staff members and volunteers do not wear artificial fingernails. Natural nail tips are less than a quarter inch long.

❑ Alcohol-based hand sanitizers are used only when hands are not visibly soiled and when running water is not available, such as during field trips or other outings.

Did you know? The 2011 *National Health and Safety Performance Standards* allows the use of alcohol-based hand sanitizers by adults and children over twenty-four months when hands are not visibly soiled. Such sanitizers can be effective and convenient. However, because they contain alcohol, they are also toxic when ingested in significant quantities. You must take precautions when storing and using them so children do not use or have access to them without supervision.

Alcohol-based hand sanitizers do not remove soil. The friction created by using soap and running water is the most effective way to remove soil from hands. Hand sanitizers can supplement but do not replace routine hand washing in child care programs.

❑ Premoistened towelettes are not used as substitutes for hand washing or alcohol-based hand sanitizers.

❑ Staff members and volunteers wash hands when they arrive at the program.

❑ Teachers and volunteers wash hands before working with a second group of children.

❑ Staff members and volunteers wash hands before and after handling food, even when food service gloves are used.

❑ Teachers and volunteers wash hands after assisting a child with nose blowing. They wash before and after giving first aid, even when gloves are used.

❑ Teachers and volunteers wash hands before and after diapering, assisting with toileting, and giving medication.

❑ Teachers and volunteers wash hands after using art and sensory materials, such as playdough, clay, and sand.

❑ Teachers and volunteers wash hands before and after involvement in water table play.

❑ Staff members and volunteers wash hands after handling animals, animal foods, and supplies.

❑ Staff members and volunteers wash hands after handling garbage.

❑ Staff members and volunteers wash hands after using the toilet.

❑ Staff members and volunteers wash hands before leaving at the end of the day.

❑ Staff members and volunteers follow the hand-washing procedure recommended by the American Academy of Pediatrics. (See appendix D in this book to review the recommended hand-washing procedure.)

Did you know? When washing your hands, be careful to clean under and around jewelry, including rings, watches, and bracelets. Jewelry is an excellent hiding place for dirt and germs. If your jewelry is too delicate to withstand frequent, vigorous hand washing, remove it while working with children.

❑ Staff members and volunteers remove gloves before washing hands.

❑ Staff members and volunteers are trained to wash hands effectively when they start working in the program and routinely throughout their term of employment/volunteerism.

❑ Staff members and volunteers are monitored for compliance with hand-washing procedures.

CHILDREN

Goal: Children practice routine hand washing to ensure they do not transmit illness and infection.

❑ Children are supported in learning and practicing regular and thorough hand washing.

Did you know? So children wash their hands thoroughly, use some teaching tricks to keep them at the sink for longer periods of time. Encourage them to keep their hands under the running water and to rub vigorously for as long as it takes to sing the alphabet or another short song. Singing a short song gives children a way to measure the time and stay engaged while they wash their hands!

❑ Infants' hands are gently washed before and after feeding.

❑ Infants' hands are gently washed after diapering.

❑ Infants' hands are gently washed after interacting with art or sensory materials or pets.

❑ Toddlers and preschoolers are required to thoroughly wash hands upon arrival, before meals, and after using the toilet or being diapered.

❑ Toddlers and preschoolers are encouraged to thoroughly wash hands after meals, before and after handling art or sensory materials, after interacting with animals, and after blowing noses or sneezing.

❑ Proper supplies for frequent, thorough hand washing are readily available.

❑ Hand-washing sinks are at child height or sturdy step stools are available so children can wash their hands independently.

❑ Alcohol-based hand sanitizers are used only when hands are not visibly soiled.

❑ Alcohol-based hand sanitizers are not used by children under twenty-four months of age.

❑ Antimicrobial soaps are not used.

Did you know? A great deal has recently been written about **antibacterial** products. It is tempting to think that a product that kills bacteria is a good buy. But in fact, these products have some hidden dangers. Several studies indicate that antibacterial products are no better than ordinary soap and water for removing bacteria. They have no impact on viruses. Some experts are also concerned about effects (Boise 2010a). The evidence that widespread use of antibacterial chemicals may be linked to cancers and other harmful health is not conclusive. But given the modest, if any, benefit of these chemicals, it's best to avoid using them on young children if possible.

❑ Premoistened towelettes are not used as substitutes for hand washing or alcohol-based hand sanitizers.

❑ Children are taught the importance of hand washing. They are taught hand-washing procedures that reduce the risk of illness and infection.

❑ Children's hand washing is supervised so it conforms to the Centers for Disease Control and Prevention's hand-washing procedure.

Standard Precautions

You are likely to come in contact with blood when working with young children. A child scrapes his knee; a child has a bloody nose; a child picks a scab from an old injury. These situations are common in child care programs. On the surface, they seem hazard-free. But some bacteria and viruses carried in blood pose a risk to children and adults in child care environments. These bacteria and viruses are known as **blood-borne pathogens**. Although the risk is small, you should minimize it by using precautions known as **standard precautions**.

The Centers for Disease Control and Prevention (CDC) requires standard precautions (which are sometimes referred to as *universal precautions*) for handling potential exposure to blood, blood-containing body fluids, and tissue discharges, such as feces and mucous, in child care environments. The standard precautions require teachers to treat all blood and blood-containing body fluids as if they are infected. You cannot know which children have potentially dangerous bacteria or viruses in their blood or bodily fluids. So you must assume that all are risky and use the same precautions in all situations. Even when you know or believe that a child is healthy, you must treat that child's blood and body fluids as if they are infected. The CDC's standard precautions are taught as part of your first aid training.

The Occupational Safety and Health Administration (OSHA) has developed standards for employers to protect employees from exposure to potentially infected blood and bodily fluids in the workplace. You can read about workplace standards in Leadership, part 6 of *Healthy Children, Healthy Lives*.

STANDARD PRECAUTIONS

Goal: We protect children and ourselves from blood-borne illnesses transmitted in blood and blood-containing body fluids.

❑ New staff members and volunteers receive training on risks associated with blood-borne pathogens. They learn appropriate precautions for use in giving first aid, diapering, and otherwise caring for young children.

❑ Staff members and volunteers receive annual training on risks associated with blood-borne pathogens. They learn appropriate precautions to use in giving first aid, diapering, and caring for young children.

❑ Single-use, nonporous gloves are readily available indoors and outdoors to avoid contact with blood.

❑ Staff members and volunteers use standard precautions during all contact with blood or blood-containing fluids.

Did you know? Many situations involving blood occur when children are playing outdoors. Unfortunately, gloves are often out of reach then. Pack a small backpack or waist pack with necessary supplies, such as gloves, to comply with standard precautions outdoors, wear the pack whenever you leave the building so safety supplies are always within reach.

❑ Surfaces that are routinely contaminated by blood or body fluids (for example, changing tables and sinks) are made of nonporous materials that can be easily cleaned and sanitized.

❑ Surfaces and materials contaminated by blood or body fluids are immediately cleaned and then sanitized. Children are kept away from the surfaces before and during **sanitizing**.

❑ Porous materials, such as rugs, carpeting, and upholstered furnishings, are cleaned and sanitized as soon as possible when they are contaminated by blood or blood-containing body fluids. Children are kept away from the contaminated area until it has been sanitized.

❑ Blood-containing materials, including diapers and bandages, are disposed of in securely sealed plastic bags.

Health Information

Child care programs collect a wide variety of information about children, their development, and their progress in the program. You can use this information to meet children's needs, to evaluate the success of your program, and to plan for program improvements.

You get to know the children in your care very well, so it may not seem important to collect much information about their health. It may seem obvious when a child is ill, and your program may not serve sick children. But young children can't always tell adults about how they feel. Adults must work together to gather information and communicate about the health needs of young children. You will need information from families and possibly from doctors, nurses, or medical practitioners for a full picture of each child's unique needs. You will also need to communicate with families about your concerns for the health of their children. Working closely with families to gather health information tells them that monitoring a young child's health is important. They see that you are devoted to their child's well-being.

Agencies that monitor and license child care programs often require specific health information to be collected and maintained. Agencies may require specific forms or types of forms. Check with your program's licensing representative to be sure you are complying with the requirements in your area.

CHILDREN'S HEALTH INFORMATION

Goal: Our program has procedures for gathering health information about children and for communicating about children's health.

❑ At the time a child is enrolled, written health information is collected. This includes name and contact information for the child's primary medical care; description of developmental variations, sensory impairments, or diagnosed disabilities; description of the child's current developmental status; current medications; special concerns, such as **allergies** or **chronic illnesses**; diet restrictions; dates of communicable illnesses; and immunization information.

Did you know? Your licensing agency or child care health consultant may provide forms for collecting children's health information. You can download a number of useful forms, like a symptom record, from the online version of Caring for Our Children: National Health and Safety Performance Standards (AAP et al. 2011). Or you can download the entire *Caring for Our Children* document. Visit the National Resource Center for Health and Safety in Child Care and Early Education website (http://nrckids.org/).

❑ Health information is reviewed with the family face-to-face at the time of enrollment.

❑ Regular observations of children's health status are added to their records.

❑ Referrals to medical practitioners are included in children's files.

❑ Communications with families about children's health are documented in their files.

❑ Meetings are scheduled regularly with families to update health information collected at the time of enrollment.

❑ Health-related files are stored confidentially. Access to files is provided only to those staff members who need it to ensure high-quality care for children.

❑ Parental consent is obtained before a child's health records are shared with anyone other than staff members caring for the child.

❑ Children's health records are routinely reviewed to identify improvement needed in health-related practices or policies.

Immunizations

Many serious illnesses can be prevented by **immunization** received during childhood. The Centers for Disease Control and Prevention (CDC), American Academy of Family Physicians (AAFP), and the American Academy of Pediatrics (AAP) have developed a recommended immunization schedule for children from birth through age eighteen that describes when healthy children should be immunized. The immunizations recommended have been demonstrated to be safe. The small risks associated are far outweighed by the potential benefits to children and society.

Many children are not adequately immunized against preventable diseases, such as diphtheria, tetanus, pertussis, poliovirus, measles, Haemophilus influenzae type b (Hib), hepatitis B, and chicken pox (varicella). The 2009 National Immunization Survey reports that only 65 percent of children living above the national poverty guideline have received their vaccinations on schedule. Only 61 percent of children living below the poverty guideline have done so (Seith and Isakson 2011). Child care programs can play an important role in helping parents maintain their children's immunization schedule by notifying families when immunizations are needed and by connecting families to immunization clinics or health care providers.

Children may not be receiving their immunizations for many reasons. Some families have religious, cultural, or philosophical objections to immunizing children. Others can't afford to go to a doctor or clinic. They may not know about community health programs for immunization. Sometimes children's immunizations have been delayed because of illness. Your licensing or regulatory agency may have requirements for how you document objections to immunizations or delays to the recommended schedule of immunizations. Check with your licensing agency or child care health consultant so your documentation meets the requirements in your area.

CHILD IMMUNIZATIONS

Goal: We support compliance with the CDC's and AAP's recommended immunization schedule for children.

❑ Children enrolled in the program are expected to be immunized as described in the immunization schedule recommended by the CDC. (See appendix E in this book to review the recommended immunization schedule.)

❑ Immunization information is collected at enrollment, before the child attends the program.

❑ Exemptions from immunization for medical, cultural, or religious reasons are documented and kept in children's files.

Did you know? Sometimes families are afraid to have their children immunized because they believe the vaccines are unsafe or may cause autism. In 1999 the AAP created the Childhood Immunization Support Program (CISP). It provides evidence-based information and education about immunizations. Share with hesitant families the useful information you'll find on the CISP website (www2.aap.org/immunization/about/programfacts.html) and on the National Network for Immunization Information website (www.immunizationinfo.org).

❑ A system is in place to notify families when scheduled immunizations are due.

❑ A system is in place to notify families when scheduled immunizations are overdue. The notification clearly explains that enrollment may be terminated if required immunizations are not obtained.

❑ When scheduled immunizations are not obtained, families must provide a documented plan for obtaining the immunizations quickly. (They can also provide a signed waiver for your files.)

❑ Families are referred to community resources if they need immunizations for their child.

Dental/Oral Health

Considerable effort must go into addressing children's oral health. As soon as they have teeth, children need consistent dental care to protect them from cavities and other dental problems. Early care develops children's healthy habits for life.

Cavities result from tooth decay caused by the buildup of plaque and acid-producing bacteria on teeth. They can be painful and can result in premature loss of teeth. Chronic dental disease is associated with other health conditions, such as diabetes, heart disease, and cancer. Most cavities can be prevented by routine and thorough toothbrushing, adequate fluoride supplements, and learning to floss. Toothbrushing is one of the first healthy habits children learn. Its benefits last a lifetime.

Children should brush their teeth at least twice each day. Two meals and some snacks each day in child care mean it's reasonable to plan for toothbrushing during the child care day. Half-day and other short programs may not provide toothbrushing. They may instead ask children to rinse their mouths with water after snacks and encourage other dental care at home.

Even when the water supply contains fluoride, toothpaste with fluoride is recommended for children age two and older. The use of toothpaste with fluoride for children younger than two is controversial. Consult the child's family for direction. Ingesting large amounts of fluoride is not recommended. Be sure to supervise children to ensure that at most only very small amounts of fluoridated toothpaste are swallowed.

DENTAL/ORAL HEALTH

Goal: We protect children's dental and oral health.

- ❑ Infant teachers clean infants' teeth with a moistened soft cloth at least once a day. With family permission, a smear of toothpaste (the size of a grain of rice) may be used.

- ❑ Children are not allowed to continue bottle feeding while sleeping. Bottles are never placed alongside sleeping children in cribs.

- ❑ Fruit juices and sugary drinks are never served in bottles.

- ❑ Water is provided throughout the day for children over six months to drink.

- ❑ Children are not allowed to continuously drink formula, milk, or juice from bottles or sippy cups.

- ❑ Children have their own age-appropriate toothbrushes labeled with their names.

- ❑ Children's toothbrushes are stored individually, do not touch other toothbrushes, and are rinsed thoroughly after each use.

❑ Fluoridated toothpaste is provided, or each family must provide fluoridated toothpaste for their child.

❑ Toothpaste is distributed on paper, in paper cups, or from individual tubes to prevent contamination of toothbrushes.

❑ Toothbrushing occurs at least twice a day. Children are encouraged to rinse their mouths with water after meals or snacks, especially those with sticky or sugary foods, such as raisins.

❑ Rinsing with water is encouraged when toothbrushing is not possible.

❑ Teachers or volunteers help toddlers and preschoolers brush their teeth after meals and snacks.

❑ Children are closely monitored during toothbrushing so it is thorough. They do not ingest much toothpaste.

Did you know? Children benefit from using fluoridated toothpastes, but eating too much fluoride can be harmful. Many people use much more toothpaste than is really needed. Use the right amount of toothpaste and supervise toothbrushing carefully. For children under two years, a smear of toothpaste equal to a grain of rice is sufficient. For children over two years of age, a pea-sized smear is adequate.

❑ Dental health is discussed in our program as an important component of health.

❑ We ask families for information about the child's dental care during enrollment.

Health Consultation

You can't be completely knowledgeable about the wide range of health and health-related situations that occur in child care programs. Health risks and healthy practices change all the time. It's a best practice to partner with a child care health consultant to support you and your program in providing the healthiest care possible.

Child care health consultants are trained in a wide range of health-related topics: child development, child care regulations, and policies and practices that affect child care programs. In some regions, child care regulations require programs to use child care health consultants. Even where regulations do not require this procedure, consulting one is a wise practice.

Your child care health consultant will be an important and valued part of your program. So it's important to make a careful decision when selecting one. Some programs are tempted to ask a parent or an acquaintance who works in health care to serve as the program's child care health consultant. But not all health professionals are suited to child care programs. You are most likely to get full value from a child care health consultant who has been carefully selected, visits regularly, and forms a true partnership with the program. The objective viewpoint offered by a trained child care health consultant is valuable to your program. A parent who uses your program or a friend or acquaintance is not as likely to be objective.

CHILD CARE HEALTH CONSULTANT

Goal: We support the health of the children in our program by using a qualified child care health consultant.

❑ Our program has an ongoing partnership with a child care health consultant. The consultant meets the qualifications described by the American Academy of Pediatrics in *Caring for Our Children: National Health and Safety Performance Standards* (AAP et al. 2011).

Did you know? If you do not currently have a child care health consultant, your licensing or regulatory agent may be able to recommend one in your area. Your local Child Care Resource and Referral Agency may have a list of child care health consultants. The American Academy of Pediatrics maintains a list of state contacts for child care health consultation online at www.healthychildcare.org/pdf/CCCCFlyer.pdf.

❑ The families served by our program know about our partnership with a child care health consultant. They have given written approval for the child care health consultant to review children's records.

❑ Our child care health consultant reviews our health-related policies and procedures at least once annually.

❑ Our child care health consultant routinely reviews at least some of the children's records to identify health and illness trends and compliance with health-related policies, including immunizations.

❑ Our child care health consultant visits the program at least monthly when infants and toddlers are served or at least quarterly when only children older than two years are served.

❑ Our child care health consultant interacts with the children and all of the adults working in the program, including teachers, cooks, and administrators.

❑ We can contact our child care health consultant between visits for advice on health-related issues.

❑ We have a system for documenting the results of the child care health consultant's visit, for example, observations, recommendations, and resources provided.

❑ We implement all or most of the child care health consultant's recommendations.

❑ Our child care health consultant arranges or provides training or resources in response to observations during the visit as needed.

Section 15

Addressing Illness and Special Health Needs of Children

Even when you carefully implement prevention routines, some illness is inevitable in child care programs. Children do not have fully developed hygiene habits, and many childhood illnesses are contagious long before symptoms appear. You must be aware of the potential symptoms of common childhood illnesses. Being alert to changes in children's behavior and other symptoms will help you pinpoint those times when action is required.

When children become ill while attending the program, you have three priorities:

1. You must minimize other children's exposure to illness.

2. The sick child must be made as comfortable as possible.

3. The child's family must be notified so appropriate medical care can be arranged.

Although most programs do not care for ill children, you will probably be asked to give medications to young children. Doing so is a serious responsibility. Although **prescription** and **over-the-counter,** or nonprescription, medications can be helpful in treating illness, they can also threaten children's health. Because of possible harmful side effects and possible dosage errors, giving medication can never be routine. It should not be taken lightly. You can give medicine safely and effectively. Use the precautions and practices described here to feel more confident about medicating children safely.

Many child care programs provide care for children with special or chronic health needs. You may care for children who have **allergies**, diabetes, epilepsy, or other **chronic illnesses** or **chronic health care needs**. While they are like other children in most ways, these children have some unique needs you should know about.

This section will address:

- Identifying illness: One of the best ways to minimize illness is to identify ill children as quickly as possible to limit other children's exposure to them.

- Illness outbreaks: Illness is inevitable, so you must be prepared to deal with outbreaks when they occur.

- Administering medications: If your program chooses to give medications, you must take precautions so it's done safely.

- Chronic illnesses or chronic health care needs: Many programs care for at least one child with a special health need, such as allergies or diabetes. Care for these children requires thoughtful consideration.

- Allergies: Children's reactions to **allergens** can be mild or severe. Always be prepared for allergic reactions, because they can occur anytime.

Identifying Illness

Despite your best efforts, children in your care will become ill. Illnesses in child care environments can be transmitted several ways: through body fluids exchanged during person-to-person contact or through droplets that land on toys, tables, or other surfaces when ill children cough or sneeze. Some microorganisms can be transmitted through the air. Chicken pox and measles viruses are transmitted that way. Unfortunately, some transmission occurs before children show signs of illness.

One of the best ways to minimize transmission is to identify children who may be ill early. Early identification limits the time that ill children are in contact with healthy children. It helps families seek medical treatment right away. But most teachers are not trained to diagnose illnesses. In fact, unless they are trained, teachers should avoid diagnosing or making guesses about childhood illnesses. So what can you do? You should become familiar with symptoms commonly associated with childhood illnesses. When you observe these symptoms, you can take precautions to minimize exposure and alert families so they can seek medical advice.

One of the commonly cited symptoms of illness is **fever**. Children's temperatures may be elevated for several reasons, not all of them illness. Fever accompanied by behavioral change is a more accurate indication of illness.

Fever alone is rarely associated with contagious illnesses, but most child care licensing regulations list fever as an exclusion criterion. Your program's **exclusion policy** must meet the criteria set by your regulatory agency. And you can include additional criteria. You must be familiar with and use the exclusion criteria described in your licensing regulations.

IDENTIFYING ILLNESS

Goal: Our program follows procedures that prevent or minimize illness outbreaks.

❑ Teachers are trained by our child care health consultant or another health professional designated by our regulatory agency to recognize potential symptoms of common childhood illnesses.

❑ Teachers are trained to recognize potential symptoms of illnesses that do not require exclusion from the program but may merit increased attention to hygiene, for example, fifth disease, mild respiratory infections, and ear infections.

❑ Teachers are trained by our child care health consultant or other agency-approved health professionals in age-appropriate techniques to monitor children's temperatures.

❑ Children are routinely observed for potential signs of illness as they enter the program each day.

❑ Families are made aware at the time of enrollment of the program's exclusion policy.

❑ The program's written exclusion policy describes the criteria that result in the exclusion of children from the program, how family members will be contacted should a child become ill while attending the program, and circumstances under which children may return to the program.

❑ The exclusion policy is consistently enforced for all children, including children of adults working in the program.

Did you know? One of the best indicators that children are ill is their inability to participate in the program. If they are not feeling well enough to play or to interact with others in typical ways, they are probably ill. This criterion may seem more subjective than an elevated temperature, but it may be a better indicator of a child's actual health.

Illness Outbreaks

Even when you use best practices for maintaining a healthy environment, young children become ill from time to time. When that happens, you need to balance the needs of ill children with the well-being of the others. Ill children should be separated from the group. They require constant supervision and a comfortable space to rest until families can arrive. The American Academy of Pediatrics (AAP) has developed an excellent table describing symptoms of common childhood illnesses as well as exclusion criteria for each. Although the AAP's list does not override your local regulations, it provides helpful guidance. The table is appendix A in the online version of *Caring for Our Children: National Health and Safety Standards* (AAP et al. 2011).

When families arrive, they need information about the ill child's symptoms. Documentation that helps them seek treatment can also help you look for trends and prevent illness outbreaks. Families usually want to know what symptoms were observed and what the exclusion requirement will be. This information helps them plan for how long the child cannot attend the program.

Sometimes you'll need to notify the families of other children that one child has become ill. You may also need to report some communicable illnesses to local authorities. Your licensing agency or local health department has guidelines stating which illnesses must be reported to agencies and/or families.

ILLNESS OUTBREAKS

Goal: We respond to illness in ways that limit the spread of illness and address the needs of ill children.

❑ We have enough adults to supervise children who become ill.

❑ We have ample space to keep children who become ill away from healthy children until families can pick up sick children.

❑ The space used to exclude ill children is comfortable and stocked with activities appropriate to the abilities of the ill children.

❑ Electronic media are never used with children who are ill.

❑ When children become ill, families receive complete instructions about criteria that children must meet to return to the program. They are also given information to help their medical provider, such as the children's symptoms.

❑ When children are diagnosed with a communicable illness, families of other children in the same environment or classroom are notified. They are provided with a description of the symptoms, when symptoms are likely to appear, and exclusion criteria.

❑ Records of illness outbreaks include the date and time of the symptoms, names of those affected, a description of the symptoms, the program's response, persons notified, and the name of the adult recording the information.

Did you know? Finding ways to notify all families of illness in the program can be challenging. Some programs use written notes that are distributed with children's take-home items. Some programs post notices in areas where families expect to look for program information, such as a program bulletin board. Programs are increasingly using e-mail to communicate with families about illness, but for this to be effective, programs must be sure all families have access to e-mail; if they don't, the program must have a second method of communication. Regardless of the delivery method, all communication about illness should be done in a way that respects confidentiality and minimizes unnecessary concern. A note posted in a hallway announcing an illness without also sharing precautionary measures and transmission facts can alarm families, even if it's not intended to.

Administering Medications

Child care programs differ in how they give children's medications. Some programs choose not to give them, so families must do so at home. Other programs give medications as part of their services to families to fully meet children's needs. The Americans with Disabilities Act (ADA) may require your program to give medications to children with certain disabilities or special health needs. You should obtain legal advice before deciding not to give medication.

Children's physicians may prescribe medications, or they may tell families to give nonprescription (over-the-counter) medications from drugstores or other stores. Medications can relieve symptoms, make children more comfortable while they heal, allow them to continue typical activities despite chronic or acute illness, and speed recovery from illness or infection. Some **chronic illnesses**, such as seizure disorders or diabetes, may require ongoing medications. Other illnesses or infections may require medication only once or for a few days or weeks.

Medications are given several ways. Pills and liquids are given orally, while other medications are applied to the skin as ointments. Some must be inhaled through nebulizers or nasal sprays. Others, like insulin and epinephrine, are injected by syringe or EpiPen. Licensing regulations may permit you to administer some but not other medications. You must be certain that staff members who are responsible for giving medication are properly trained to do so.

Your licensing regulations cover the giving of medications. You must adhere to these requirements. You can also put policies and procedures in place that exceed the minimum licensing regulations. Check your licensing regulations carefully. In some areas, over-the-counter medications are treated exactly the same as **prescription medications**, but in others, they are treated differently.

MEDICATION POLICY

Goal: Our medication policies meet the needs of children and families and minimize the risk of error during medication administration.

❑ Families are given written notice of medication-related policies when they enroll.

❑ Medication policies are reviewed with families annually.

❑ Our policies describe the prescription and over-the-counter (nonprescription) medications that can be given. They also specify how medications are to be given.

❑ Over-the-counter (nonprescription) medications are treated the same way as prescription medications. They are given only with written direction from children's physicians.

❑ Our medication policies require that the first dose of any medication cannot be given in our program.

❑ Our medication policies describe the conditions under which medication will be given and the adults responsible for administering medications.

❑ Our medication policies were developed with the advice of a child care health consultant. They are regularly reviewed by the consultant.

❑ Our medication policies reflect the practices described here under Medication Procedures.

Did you know? You may think that it is easy to determine what a medication is, but it's more challenging than you think. Some licensing authorities consider sunscreen an over-the-counter medication. Some view diaper ointment as an over-the-counter medication. Other places, insect repellent is treated as an over-the-counter medication. Check your licensing regulations carefully to be sure you know what is and is not considered a medication. Also review the approvals needed for their use.

MEDICATION PROCEDURES

Goal: Our medication procedures meet the needs of children and families. They minimize medication errors.

❑ Only adult staff members who are trained to give medications may do so.

❑ Training in giving medication is provided by the program's child care health consultant or other health professionals designated by the licensing agency.

❑ Staff members are trained in several methods of medication administration, such as oral, topical, and injections, including the use of EpiPens.

❑ Only designated staff members give medication to children, except in emergencies when designated staff members are not available. Substitutes, volunteers, and temporary employees are never permitted to give medication, even if they are trained to do so.

❑ Families complete a communication log or form to notify us when medications are required. The form or log includes
  ❑ name of child
  ❑ name of medication
  ❑ time(s) when medication is to be given
  ❑ dosage
  ❑ potential known side effects of medication

❑ All medications, prescription and nonprescription, are kept in their original containers with intact labels.

❏ Staff members give prescription medications only when their labels include
- ❏ patient's name
- ❏ name of medication
- ❏ date medication was prescribed
- ❏ name of physician prescribing medication
- ❏ medication's expiration date
- ❏ strength and dosage of medication prescribed
- ❏ directions for storing medication

❏ A procedure is in place for giving medications. It includes
- ❏ checking the name of the child the medication is intended for
- ❏ reading the label
- ❏ checking directions from the physician
- ❏ rechecking the medication label before administering
- ❏ rechecking the child who is receiving medication to see the name on the medication label matches the child's

❏ Staff members give each medication individually to minimize chance that medications will be confused.

❏ Staff members give medications in well-lit places where they can focus solely on giving medication.

❏ Medication is given by one adult staff member observed by a second adult staff member.

❏ Staff members wash hands before and after giving medications.

❏ Our procedure for giving medications includes maintaining a medication log. The log includes
- ❏ name of child
- ❏ name of medication
- ❏ dosage
- ❏ date and time medications were given
- ❏ full name of person giving medication

Did you know? If you want to update your medication log, check first with your child care health consultant, who may have excellent forms for use in your program. A sample form is also included in the online version of *Caring for Our Children: National Health and Safety Performance Standards* (AAP et al. 2011), appendix AA (http://nrckids.org/).

❑ Medications are stored out of the reach of children in a locked cabinet or container.

❑ Medications requiring refrigeration are stored in a locked container inside the refrigerator.

❑ Medications are given only according to the prescription label directions and physician's instructions, even if families request otherwise.

❑ Medications are given only when specific direction is provided by the child's physician. Medications are never given "as needed."

❑ Liquid medications are given using standard measuring spoons or droppers designed for medication. Tableware spoons are never used.

❑ Medication errors are reported immediately to children's families. Emergency procedures are implemented if signs of adverse reactions occur.

Did you know? Administering medication is a serious responsibility that requires attention to small details. When errors are made in the administering of medications—giving a medication to the wrong child, giving a child the wrong medication, giving the wrong dosage of a medication, or giving a medication too frequently or too infrequently—serious consequences can result. If a medication error occurs, it is important to report the error immediately rather than to wait for a side effect to occur.

Chronic Illnesses or Chronic Health Care Needs

The U.S. Department of Health and Human Services estimates that 14 percent of children have **chronic illnesses** or **chronic health care needs** (Donoghue and Kraft 2010). Millions of these children attend child care programs, where their chronic medical needs must be met. Advances in medical care, early interventions, and other treatments have made it possible for more children with chronic illnesses or chronic health care needs to participate in typical child care programs. Chronic illnesses and chronic health care needs are conditions that are expected to continue over a long period of time or over the child's lifetime. For example, diabetes is a chronic illness that requires special health care. Some chronic health care needs are not illness but do require special health care attention. For example, allergies are chronic health care needs that are not illnesses.

Other health care needs that are not chronic may require special accommodations while the child participates in the program. For example, a child may be recuperating from an operation and require special therapy or activities. Research consistently supports including children with chronic or other health needs in child care programs. Doing so benefits all children and their families.

Children with diagnosed chronic or other health needs must have care plans in place. In some states, these are referred to as Individual Health Care Plans (IHCP). Care plans help you understand children's needs and your responsibilities in providing care. Usually care plans are developed by children's health care providers, therapists, and families and include

- medical information about the child's health status

- details describing medications, treatments, or other medical procedures that may be required

- modifications in daily routines that may be needed to accommodate the child's needs

- responses that may be needed in emergency situations, including symptoms or signals to watch for

Even if you do not have children with chronic and special health needs in your program now, you should have policies in place that conform with the procedures in this checklist.

CHRONIC AND SPECIAL HEALTH NEEDS

Goal: Our program meets the needs of children with chronic illnesses or chronic and special health needs.

❑ When children with health needs enroll in the program, the family and the child's health care provider supply a care plan for the child.

❑ A care plan is developed as soon as possible when a child already enrolled in the program is diagnosed with a chronic or other health care need.

❑ Before the child's first day of care or as soon as the care plan is developed, we meet with family members and health care providers (if possible) to review the care plan and ask and answer any questions about it.

Did you know? Responsibility for providing care for children with chronic or other health care needs can initially seem overwhelming. Many professionals stand by to help you understand your role and to support you in meeting children's needs. Be open to asking questions and seeking support. Families and health professionals do not expect you to have all the answers or to know a great deal about medical conditions and situations. But you need to be honest and open with them about what you do know and about what you need to know. Doing so helps you form true partnerships and best meet children's needs.

❑ Staff members meet with family members and health care professionals (if possible) to review the care plan. This is done regularly and as needed when the child's condition changes.

❑ Our program obtains written permission from families to seek information from children's health care providers about children with chronic or other health care needs.

❑ Staff members receive training from our child care health consultant or appropriate health professionals on implementing the care plan, giving medications, and responding to emergencies that may occur associated with children's chronic or other health care needs.

❑ Staff members receive training about modifications that may be needed in the environment or activities to accommodate a child's chronic or other health care needs.

❑ Staff members meet regularly with family members to discuss the child's development. Successes and challenges associated with modifications made to meet the child's needs are reviewed.

❑ Staff members cooperate fully with therapists and others who work with the family.

❑ Our program has plans for responding to emergencies that may occur with children's chronic or other health care needs. For example, staff members know how to respond to asthma attacks or seizures.

Allergies

The Asthma and Allergy Foundation of America (2011) estimates that one in five people in the United States reacts to at least one **allergen**. There are many kinds of allergies. They can be grouped into such categories such as respiratory or airborne allergies (animal dander, hay fever), skin allergies (poison ivy, latex), food and drug allergies (peanuts, milk, penicillin), and insect allergies (bee stings, dust mites). Allergies cannot be cured, but most can be managed and treated. Allergic reactions can be mild (a runny nose or a slight rash) or severe (lowered blood pressure, difficulty breathing, even death).

Anaphylaxis is a life-threatening allergic reaction. It often occurs with no warning and within minutes of contact with an allergen. It requires an immediate response. Food allergies (especially nuts), insect stings, latex allergies, and reactions to medications are its most common triggers. Although anaphylaxis is very rare, occurring in only thirty of one hundred thousand persons, it is critical that you are prepared when the reaction occurs (Donoghue and Kraft 2010).

ALLERGIES

Goal: We are prepared to respond to allergic reactions.

❑ Staff members are trained to recognize the signs of allergic reactions by our child care health consultant or another health professional designated by our licensing regulations.

❑ All staff members are trained and certified in first aid, including response to allergic reactions, anaphylaxis, and use of EpiPens.

❑ Staff members communicate with families when they see any signs of an allergic reaction.

❑ Our program requires information from the child's health care provider about known allergies, allergens, symptoms and severity of reactions, and medications used to prevent and treat reactions.

❑ Our program has a system for informing all staff members, including substitute and temporary staff members, about preventing exposure to allergens, signs of allergic reactions, and responses to allergic reactions.

❑ Our program has eliminated as many known allergens as possible.

❑ Our program has minimized exposure to allergens when eliminating them isn't possible. For example, a child allergic to milk may be served an alternate such as soy milk or rice-based milk. Milk and milk products are kept away from the child who is allergic.

Did you know? When you develop policies to minimize known allergens, be careful about what you promise. For example, it is difficult, and perhaps impossible, to provide an environment that is 100 percent "peanut free"; you cannot, after all, completely control every person who visits your program. It makes more sense to call your efforts "peanut safe."

❑ When new families enroll in the program, they are told about known allergens and the precautions necessary to protect the health of children with allergies.

❑ Staff members enforce precautions developed to protect children from known allergens.

Did you know? It may be tempting to make exceptions to rules meant to help protect children from allergens. For example, you may have a peanut-safe environment but want to allow peanut butter sandwiches on a field trip. Making such exceptions only confuses the situation for everyone. It also puts a child at great risk. Once you create your policy, stick to it. Consistency and clarity are the best approach to protecting children's health.

Section 16

Environment

Young children are particularly susceptible to their environment. Because they are still growing and developing, they need a healthy environment to support optimum growth and development. They can't fully protect themselves from environmental hazards through good choices or excellent hygiene habits, because they are just learning skills such as hand washing and toileting. The child care environment can have a positive influence on children's health and their development of healthy habits. This section will help you establish policies and practices to make the physical environment a positive, safe one for the children you serve.

Young children need little encouragement to be messy. Their explorations of interactions with food, art materials, sand and water, and each other naturally result in spills, smears, and sticky handprints. You encourage messy play, and you're also responsible for routine housekeeping to keep the environment neat and orderly and to reduce the spread of germs.

Young children are just learning to care for their environment independently. Their newly developing hygiene habits contribute to your challenges in maintaining the environment. Cleanliness is essential to protect children's health and to appeal to their families. Families make judgments about children's quality of care based on what they see in your program. Many families say that cleanliness is the most important factor in deciding on one child care program over another.

Cleanliness is very important in maintaining a safe environment for children. Make sure that the cleaning products and methods you use are safe for children and support their healthy development. Health and early childhood professionals and parents are increasingly concerned about young children's exposure to chemicals like sanitizers and disinfectants. As a result, many people are seeking out green products for use around children. Throughout this section, you will see references to the use of the term *green products*. Green products have a reduced impact on human health and the environment. No regulations exist to monitor a company's use of the terms *green*, *natural*, and *safe*. Effective green cleaning products are free of irritants and toxic chemicals that have been linked to long- and short-term health risks. They often contain no or few fragrances, because these have been linked to **asthma** or other respiratory risks. You can identify green cleaning products by consulting Green Seal, a nonprofit organization that evaluates such products. The Green Seal website is a helpful resource for locating green cleaning products: www.greenseal.org.

Even when your environment is clean, other potential dangers need to be avoided or minimized. You can guard children's health by minimizing their exposure to environmental hazards like air pollutants, contaminants, **lead**, and contaminated drinking water. All of these have potentially harmful effects on children's immediate and long-term health.

This section will address:

- Cleaning, sanitizing, and disinfecting: Children, like adults, grow and develop best in an environment that is clean and minimizes the spread of illness and infection. Routine cleaning, sanitizing, and disinfecting practices ensure a healthy environment for children and adults.

- Diapering and diaper-changing areas: Caring for children who are not yet using the toilet requires some unique practices to ensure health and safety.

- Toilet use and toilet areas: Young children are learning to use the toilet but still require support to ensure health and safety. For example, children using the toilet require supervision and may need reminders to wash hands after toilet use.

Cleaning, Sanitizing, and Disinfecting

You may find that the words *cleaning*, *sanitizing*, and *disinfecting* are used interchangeably by many of your colleagues. Each of these terms actually means something different. *Cleaning* removes debris so sanitizing and disinfecting agents can do the work of killing germs. Surfaces need to be cleaned before they can be sanitized or disinfected.

Sanitizing uses a sanitizer solution (such as a bleach-and-water solution of one tablespoon of bleach to one gallon of cool water) or the application of heat (AAP et al. 2011). For example, dishes or laundry can be sanitized by cleaning and the use of very hot water (over 150 degrees Fahrenheit). Sanitizing is usually required on surfaces where children eat and on any items that are mouthed by children. Sanitizing kills many, but not all, germs.

Disinfecting requires the use of agents specifically rated to kill most germs. Many programs believe they are disinfecting when they use the same bleach-and-water solution used for sanitizing. Bleach-and-water solutions used as disinfecting agents require a higher concentration of bleach than those used as sanitizers (one-half to three-quarters cup of bleach to one gallon of cool water) (AAP et al. 2011). Disinfecting is usually reserved for surfaces in bathrooms and places where diapers are changed. Your licensing regulations may require that you use disinfectants elsewhere too. Disinfectants are typically very strong. They pose health risks to children, so you need to understand if they're required and when they must be used.

CLEANING, SANITIZING, AND DISINFECTING

Goal: We protect children's health by keeping classroom materials and surfaces clean. We minimize germs to protect children from harmful chemicals.

❑ The program cleans only with soap and water or green cleaning products that have been screened and listed on the Green Seal website.

❑ Our cleaning, sanitizing, and disinfecting schedule reflects the frequency guidelines in *Caring for Our Children: National Health and Safety Performance Standards* (AAP et al. 2011). (See appendix K in this book to review the frequency guidelines.)

Did you know? Once you create a cleaning, sanitizing, and disinfecting schedule for your program, you will need to take the next steps and assign duties. You may also want to make a checkoff list for each task. Daily, weekly, and monthly checklists are helpful.

❑ Our program separates clean toys and materials from those needing cleaning and/or sanitizing (for example, mouthed toys, soiled cots, used towels).

❑ Our program uses disinfectants only when our cleaning schedule and regulatory agencies require us to. Disinfectants are EPA registered.

❑ Staff members are trained to mix and use cleaning, sanitizing, and disinfecting solutions.

❑ Staff members mix and prepare cleaning, sanitizing, and disinfecting solutions according to the manufacturer's directions. They protect children and adults by mixing solutions away from them and food. They wear protective gloves, masks, and safety glasses or goggles.

❑ Cleaning, sanitizing, and disinfecting solutions are kept in a locked storage area away from the children.

❑ Cleaning, sanitizing, and disinfecting solutions are used only according to the label directions. **Dwell time** and removal of residual after dwell time are observed.

❑ While supervising them, teachers ensure that children stay away from areas where chemicals (including bleach) are being used, during use and during dwell time.

Did you know? One of the easiest ways to keep children away from surfaces during dwell time is to sanitize just before they head outdoors or before naptime. Children are engaged in other activities while toys, door handles, and drinking fountains dry. You can also disinfect at the end of the day after children have left the program. Many providers find this the safest and most efficient time to sanitize and disinfect.

Diapering and Diaper-Changing Areas

Diapering is frequently part of the daily care-giving routine. Most children younger than three years, and some older than three years, require diapering. They are still learning to use the toilet independently. The age at which a child learns to use the toilet and no longer requires diapering varies greatly based on the child's maturity and the family's preferences. You will work closely with the families in your program to determine when children are ready to transition from diapers to using the toilet.

When you diaper children, your goal is to assist them with their soiled diapers and to return them to play feeling fresh and clean. Inevitably, you deal with body fluids that can carry disease-transmitting germs. Feces also can carry pathogens, so precautions are required there too. Follow the recommendations in this checklist to protect the health of everyone in your program: you, the child you are changing, and the other children you care for.

Pay attention to where you do diapering and how you change diapers. Diaper-changing areas are used often, usually by more than one child. Select materials and cleaners carefully, and clean and sanitize these areas thoroughly. You may change diapers many, many times each day. Like washing your hands, diapering can become almost automatic. It's easy to become complacent about this process because you do it so often. Following the entire diapering procedure each and every time is essential to maintain your and the children's healthy environment.

DIAPERING AND DIAPER-CHANGING AREAS

Goal: Our program uses safe diapering policies and practices to protect the health of children.

❑ A designated diaper-changing area is used.

❑ The diaper-changing area has nonporous, easy-to-clean surfaces, nearby running water, handy storage for diapering and cleaning supplies, and a lip of at least six inches to prevent children from rolling off the surface. It is positioned so teachers can easily supervise other children while diapering.

Did you know? Some diapering or changing tables come equipped with safety straps. And in some areas use of these straps may be required by the regulatory agency. Safety straps can be helpful in preventing children from rolling off changing tables, but they do not eliminate your need to stay within reach of children at all times. If your changing table has safety straps, you will need to clean and sanitize them thoroughly. Safety straps are excellent hiding places for soil and germs.

❑ The diaper-changing table is used by only one group of children.

❑ All teachers are trained in proper diapering procedures during **orientation** and training.

❑ The program's child care consultant observes diaper-changing practices regularly for compliance with diapering procedures.

❑ The diaper-changing area is cleaned before and after use.

❑ Diapering supplies are stored to prevent contamination. They are nearby but do not touch the diapering surface.

❑ Diapering supplies are ready before a child is brought to the diapering area.

❑ Teachers wash hands before and after diapering.

❑ Children's hands are gently washed after diapering.

❑ Teachers follow the diaper-changing procedure in *Caring for Our Children: National Health and Safety Performance Standards* (AAP et al. 2011). (See appendix C in this book to review the diaper-changing procedure.)

❑ Diaper-changing procedures are posted so they are clearly visible while diapering.

❑ Children are never left unattended during diapering.

❑ Teachers document all diapering and communicate it to families each day.

❑ Teachers communicate with families immediately if diapering suggests illness or infection, such as diarrhea or bloody stools.

Did you know? If your program provides diapering for children older than preschoolers, you need to think carefully about a diaper-changing area for them. Older children deserve privacy during diapering, and they often cannot be lifted onto typical changing tables. Work carefully with your child care health consultant and children's families to create a changing area that fits the health and safety needs of children and your program.

Toilet Use and Toilet Areas

Learning to use the toilet is an important developmental milestone. For young children, this skill comes with physical maturation, awareness, emotional security, practice, and encouragement. If you care for very young children, you will need to work closely with families to determine when their children are ready for toilet learning. Find out how the transition from diapers to toilet is being handled at home. Children more easily master this skill when their environment supports their independence. If you work with children who have already moved from diapers to toilet, you still need to be involved in their use of the toilet and toilet areas. Very few children become completely independent in their toileting and hygiene routines (such as hand washing) until they are kindergarten age.

In the early years, children are learning to use the toilet independently and to be responsible for their own hygiene. They must learn to use the toilet, wash their hands, and return to play without increasing their own exposure to germs or exposing others to their germs. Children must rely on you to provide supplies and a setting that supports independence. You need to support their emerging skills and encourage their attempts. Sometimes you need to step in with additional help. As they get older, they may want more privacy, and that makes supervision and support more challenging for you.

TOILET USE AND TOILET AREAS

Goal: We protect children's health as they learn toileting.

❑ Toilets are located away from food preparation or food service.

❑ Toilets for children are child sized. If they are not, we provide very sturdy, nonporous step stools so children can use toilets without being lifted on and off.

❑ Sinks are located next to the toilet area. These sinks are not used for food preparation. Liquid soap, running water (between 60 degrees Fahrenheit and 120 degrees Fahrenheit), single-use towels or air dryers, and trash cans are available.

❑ Preschool- and toddler-age children are supervised by sight and sound while they are using toilets.

❑ The day is organized so children can use the toilet alone or in very small groups. The number of children in the toilet area never exceeds the number of toilets available.

❑ Children wash their hands thoroughly after toileting and before returning to play.

❏ Children are encouraged to be as independent as possible during toileting. They are actively supervised to maintain hygiene.

❏ Toilet areas are cleaned on schedule and as needed during the day. We make sure that the toileting area is clean.

❏ Teachers tell families about any changes in a child's toilet habits that suggest illness or infection.

Did you know? Young children need frequent reminders to use the toilet. Even long after they have moved on from diapers, they can easily become absorbed in play and forget to respond to their bodies' cues that it is time to use the toilet. Make a special effort to regularly remind children to use the toilet. Look for signs of irritability or fidgeting that signal that children may need toilet breaks. Help them leave their activities for a few minutes to use the toilet.

Section *17*

Environmental Health

Environmental health encompasses elements in the indoor and outdoor environment that have positive or negative impacts on people. Environmental health includes the quality of air, water, and ground and substances that may be present in each of these, such as pests or contaminants.

The impact of the environment on our health is important to everyone. It is especially important to children. They are very susceptible to environmental influences because their growing bodies are more affected by contaminants and toxins than adults'. They do not fully understand the dangers of some substances and may use their senses to explore them. For example, children may put sand from the sand box in their mouths, something adults would never do. Most early childhood teachers take great pride in creating warm and engaging environments for children. Carefully keeping the environment free of contaminants is another way to create the best possible environment for young children.

Some contaminants and toxins are obvious, for example, cleaners, lawn care products, and cigarette smoke. Others may be less obvious but equally potentially dangerous. For example, everyday dust and dirt carried into the environment on boots and shoes can damage children who play and breathe very close to the floor.

This section will address:

- Air quality: The quality of the indoor and outdoor air that children (and adults) breathe affects their growth and development.

- Pest management: Pay attention to the presence of pests, such as mice or cockroaches, in or around the child care environment. You must balance the risks associated with the pests and those associated with pest-reducing chemicals.

- Body-care and hygiene products: You may use many hand soaps, sunscreens, insect repellents, and other products while caring for children. You must choose wisely so they benefit children's health.

- Contaminants: **Lead**, **asbestos**, **volatile organic compounds**, and other contaminants may be present in the environment. These toxins must be managed to protect children's health.

Air Quality

Everyone is affected by air quality. Children are more susceptible to negative impact than adults because they breathe faster, their lungs are immature, and they are closer to the ground, where many toxins accumulate. Children and adults who are sensitive to respiratory influences, such as those with **asthma**, are at greater risk. Outdoor air quality can be compromised by natural and manufactured pollutants. For example, pollen, a naturally occurring airborne substance, can be irritating to many children and adults. Similarly, the fumes from industrial processing can contain harmful irritants and toxic chemicals.

Indoor air quality is often worse than outdoor air quality because **allergens**, pollutants, fumes, and toxins can accumulate in the space. Good indoor air quality requires plenty of circulating air and no chemicals that produce fumes (Boise 2010b). It's easy to improve indoor air quality. For example, you can forbid smoking and **secondhand** and **thirdhand smoke**. Many regulatory agencies require child care environments to be smoke-free. While these requirements may not extend to secondhand and thirdhand smoke, the dangers of these exposures are increasingly well documented.

INDOOR AIR QUALITY

Goal: We protect children's health by minimizing their exposure to indoor, airborne pollutants and irritants.

❑ Smoking is prohibited at all times in or around the **facility**, within sight of the children, and in all program-related vehicles.

❑ Staff members and volunteers are aware of the dangers of thirdhand smoke. They are free of cigarette odors on their clothing, skin, and hair while working with children.

❑ Families are asked about children's sensitivities to respiratory irritants, such as **allergies** to mold, asthma, dust, or dander, when they enroll.

❑ The program has a well-maintained, filtered ventilation system with fresh air exchange.

❑ Children who are sensitive to animal allergens like dander are not exposed to animals that produce them.

❑ Children and adults wash their hands after interacting with animals.

❑ The facility is monitored monthly for mold, mildew, and insects (such as cockroaches), which can trigger respiratory problems for children.

❑ Cloth toys, fabrics, and bedding are laundered in hot water (over 140 degrees Fahrenheit) to kill dust mites.

❑ The facility has been tested for radon, high levels of carbon monoxide, and formaldehyde. It is retested every three years. If high levels of these substances are detected, we have a plan to lessen them.

❑ Candles and air and carpet fresheners are never used in the program.

❑ Rough walk-off mats are located at each entrance.

❑ Adults remove their shoes when entering areas where infants and toddlers play.

Did you know? Is your program a shoe-free environment? Many programs serving infants and toddlers keep floors clean and free from outdoor dirt by enforcing a shoe-free policy. In these programs, teachers, families, and classroom visitors remove their shoes before entering when children are present. Some teachers keep a separate pair of shoes for wear exclusively in the environment to avoid tracking substances into the space. If you change to a shoe-free environment, consider a few aids for parents and visitors. A bench outside the space where adults can sit to remove shoes is much appreciated. Some programs also provide paper booties so adults can cover rather than remove their shoes. Baskets for clean and dirty booties can be placed near a bench, or a pocket chart labeled with families' names can be hung near the door so families can reuse gently worn booties until new are needed.

❑ Carpets and rugs in children's areas are vacuumed daily. Our vacuum cleaner has a HEPA filter.

❑ Air-conditioning units and other ventilation equipment are free from debris, such as leaves.

OUTDOOR AIR QUALITY

Goal: We protect children from exposure to outdoor airborne pollutants and irritants.

❑ Staff members monitor outdoor air quality for pollution and pollen count, as measured by health experts.

❑ Children do not spend time outdoors when health officials declare that it is unhealthy to do so.

❑ A policy is in place and enforced that prevents vehicles from idling within fifty feet of the facility's doors and windows if the car is on the program's property.

❑ Signs are posted that remind drivers of the no-idle policy.

❑ Use of leaf blowers, lawn mowers, and weed cutters is prohibited when children are present.

Did you know? Work closely with your landscape vendor to arrange times for lawn mowing, leaf blowing, and other maintenance when children are not typically using the outdoor play area, for example, early morning, naptime, or late afternoon. Remember to close windows when outdoor maintenance is under way.

Pest Management

No one wants to think of a child care environment as harboring pests like mice or cockroaches. But anyplace where food is stored, crumbs abound, and other appealing discoveries are left behind by young children is very attractive to pests. You may not regularly encounter them, but pests can only be controlled with routine maintenance.

Several methods of pest management can be used. Some are quite simple, such as cleaning food preparation and storage areas, fixing water leaks, and sealing holes to keep pests from entering the facility. Others are more complex and can involve the use of a professional vendor or the application of **pesticides**. Many programs are adopting **integrated pest management** (IPM). IPM is the process of addressing pest problems in a way that is least disruptive to human health and the environment. IPM involves monitoring pests and eliminating pest habitats, and it requires working closely with your facility's staff members and vendors to determine the healthiest, most effective way to reduce pests (Boise 2010a). One of IPM's goals is to protect children and adults from harmful chemicals. Nonchemical treatments, such as removing habitats or cleaning with soapy water, can be as effective as the use of chemical pesticides.

PEST MANAGEMENT

Goal: Our program uses pesticides to manage pests and protect children from unnecessary health risks.

❑ We use a policy that describes when and how pesticides will be used safely at the facility.

❑ Holes in filters, screens, door seals, and insulation are repaired, preventing pests from getting in and reducing the need for pesticides.

❑ Pipes and hoses entering the facility are inspected monthly, and their seals are repaired as needed, preventing pests from getting in and reducing the need for pesticides.

❑ We keep records of nonchemical treatments to document our program's efforts to reduce pests.

❑ We keep records of pesticide use that include what pesticide was used, when and where it was applied, and by whom.

❑ Pesticides are not applied when children will be present within the next forty-eight hours.

❑ Families are notified when pesticides are scheduled to be applied.

Did you know? Your licensing or regulatory agencies may require you to notify families whenever pesticides are used at the facility. Even if you are not required to do this, it's a good practice to follow. If you do need to give notice, be sure you comply with all of the requirements, including what information is given and when you must give it. For example, you may be required to give notice of pesticide use forty-eight hours before it is applied.

❑ Signs are posted in the area where pesticides, including weed killers, have been used.

❑ Surfaces and materials are cleaned and fabric materials are laundered after pesticides are used and before children return.

❑ Our program follows local regulations on pesticide use.

❑ Our program uses only EPA-approved pesticides. They are applied as directed on the label. We insist that contractors do the same.

❑ Our program uses certified organic weed killers outdoors, as directed on the label. We do not allow children to use the areas where weed killers have been applied for twenty-four hours after the application.

❑ We have written agreements on file with contractors or outside parties, including volunteers, who maintain the facility. They agree to follow our program's policies on the use of pesticides.

Body-Care and Hygiene Products

Body-care and hygiene products include hand soaps, ointments, wipes, lotions (including sunscreens), and toothpastes used for cleansing, comfort, or cosmetic purposes. These are most often not prescribed. They are manufactured with few regulations and little consideration for short- and long-term health effects.

Body-care and hygiene products are marketed as goods that protect and maintain health. Some of them do play roles in overall wellness. For example, sunscreens are important in protecting skin from ultraviolet light. But some sunscreens contain chemicals with potentially harmful effects. Children's growing bodies and high skin-to-body-weight ratio put them at unique risk to absorb harmful chemicals. Choose products that do not contain these.

Antibacterial ingredients are often included in hand soaps and lotions because they are believed to prevent the spread of illness or infection. However, according to the EPA, research increasingly indicates that many of these chemicals can have serious long-term effects that are potentially more serious for young children, whose bodies are not fully developed.

Teachers can screen the safety of body-care and hygiene products by looking them up on the Environmental Working Group's (EWG's) Skin Deep Cosmetics Database (www.ewg.org /skindeep).

Your area's licensing regulations may address the use of body-care and hygiene products specifically or consider these products nonprescription medications. Be aware of any requirements for using these products, and consult your licensing regulations. For example, some licensing agencies require parent or even physician approval before lotions like sunscreens, insect repellents, or diaper creams can be used. Your program can choose to protect children further by creating policies and practices more stringent than those described in the licensing regulations.

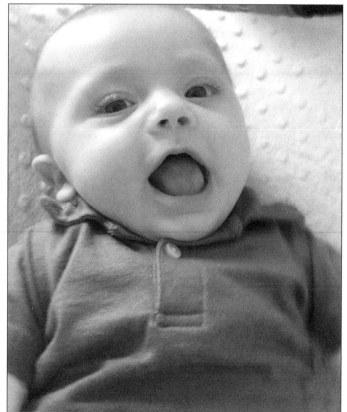

BODY-CARE AND HYGIENE PRODUCTS

Goal: We use safe body-care and hygiene products on children.

❑ The body-care and hygiene products, including hand soaps, used in our program do not contain antibacterial ingredients.

❑ Hand sanitizers used on field trips and other occasions when hand washing is not practical are alcohol based and not antibacterial.

❑ Families must give specific written permission before staff members apply lotions, sprays, or other body-care and hygiene products to children's skin. This does not include hand soap.

❑ Only products rated low hazard on the EWG's Skin Deep Cosmetics Database (www.ewg.org /skindeep) are used on children. Families are aware of this policy.

❑ Body-care and hygiene products are never sprayed directly on children. Items that are available only as sprays are applied to the teacher's hand away from the children then applied to their skin.

❑ Families test body-care and hygiene products on children at home before sending them for use in the program.

❑ If insect repellents are used, they contain less than 30 percent **DEET.** They are not used on children younger than two months and are used on children under six months of age only with a physician's permission.

❑ Oil of lemon and eucalyptus products are not used as insect repellents on children under three years of age.

Did you know? Protecting children from biting insects can be challenging. First, minimize insects by eliminating standing water and other breeding grounds. Mosquito and tick bites can be dangerous, so you may decide to use insect repellents at certain times of the year. Avoid using aerosol sprays. Use a pump dispenser, and spray the repellent into your own hand, then apply it to the child. Preschoolers and younger children should not apply their own insect repellent.

Contaminants

Dangerous chemicals or other substances in child care facilities can have negative impacts on children's immediate and long-term health. Some of these contaminants are easy to detect, while others are not. One of the most commonly recognized environmental hazards is **lead**. Lead is a mineral that used to be routinely used in paint and plumbing. In the 1970s, exposure to lead was recognized as a danger to children's cognitive development and overall health. Since 1978, paints can no longer contain lead. Older facilities may still contain risks from lead in paint. The soil surrounding older facilities may have accumulated lead residue from car exhaust. If your facility's plumbing was installed before 1986, the pipes may leach lead into your water supply.

Another risk of exposure to lead comes from children's toys. Toys manufactured in the United States do not contain lead-based paints. This is not true of all toys and children's products manufactured outside the United States.

Asbestos is another commonly recognized contaminant. Before the 1970s, asbestos was used in insulation and many products like floor and ceiling tiles. It is no longer used to make new building materials, but it can still be found in older facilities. If undisturbed, asbestos is relatively safe. However, exposed or disturbed asbestos can present a life-threatening health hazard.

More recently, **volatile organic compounds**, or VOCs, have come to the attention of educators and families. Volatile organic compounds are found in plastics and paints. They can be avoided by choosing low-VOC or VOC-free products.

LEAD

Note: If your facility was constructed after 1978 and its plumbing was installed after 1986, it is likely to present minimal risk of exposure to lead.

Goal: Our program follows practices to minimize children's exposure to lead.

❑ Our facility was constructed after 1978.

❑ Our facility has been tested, and no lead exposure was found. If lead paint was detected, it is not exposed. The paint is covered by low-VOC paint, or our program is using a lead-safe painting contractor to address the exposed lead paint.

❑ Our water has been tested, and no lead has been detected. If lead was found in the water, we are using a carbon filter system or reverse osmosis system to remove lead or using only bottled water for drinking, cooking, and cleaning.

❑ Our facility is located away from highways and roads with heavy traffic.

❑ The soil around our facility has been tested for lead deposits from vehicle emissions.

❑ Toys bought for use in our program do not contain lead-based paint.

Did you know? Buying toys for the program can be one of the fun tasks associated with working with children. Although it may be tempting and budget friendly, refrain from purchasing or accepting donations of secondhand toys. You will not have access to recall information, damage history, or warranties. Check with the vendors you use for toy purchases to be sure that toys used in the program are lead-free. Reputable vendors should be willing to certify that their products are free of lead paint to earn your business.

ASBESTOS

Note: If the facility was constructed after 1986, risk of hazards from asbestos is minimal.

Goal: Our program's practices minimize children's exposure to asbestos.

❑ A certified asbestos inspector has tested our facility, and no asbestos exposure was detected. If asbestos was detected, the program has contracted with a licensed abatement firm to properly remove the asbestos. Methods specified in the Asbestos Hazard Emergency Response Act (AHERA) have been used. After the asbestos has been removed, regular rein-spections are conducted by a certified asbestos inspector six months later and every three years thereafter. If removal of asbestos is not recommended, we have a management plan for periodic surveillance, reinspection, and maintenance (including cleaning) of asbestos materials to protect children from exposure.

❑ Families are notified during enrollment or when asbestos is discovered, even when such materials are located in areas not routinely used by children.

OTHER CONTAMINANTS

Goal: We protect children from exposure to contaminants.

❑ Only wall paints with no VOCs are used.

❑ Wall paint is applied when children are not present.

❑ Plastic containers are never used to heat, boil, cook, or microwave food or drinks.

❑ Plastics used by children are free from phthalates, PVCs, chlorine, plasticizer, and BPA, ensured by recycling codes 1, 2, 4, or 5. Plastic items with recycling codes 3, 6, and 7 are never used.

Did you know? Heating plastic containers releases any dangerous VOC that may be present, even in small quantities. When you heat baby foods, use warm water rather than the microwave. When a microwave is used to heat children's food, use nonplastic dishes like glass bowls. You can transfer the food to plastic dishes after heating.

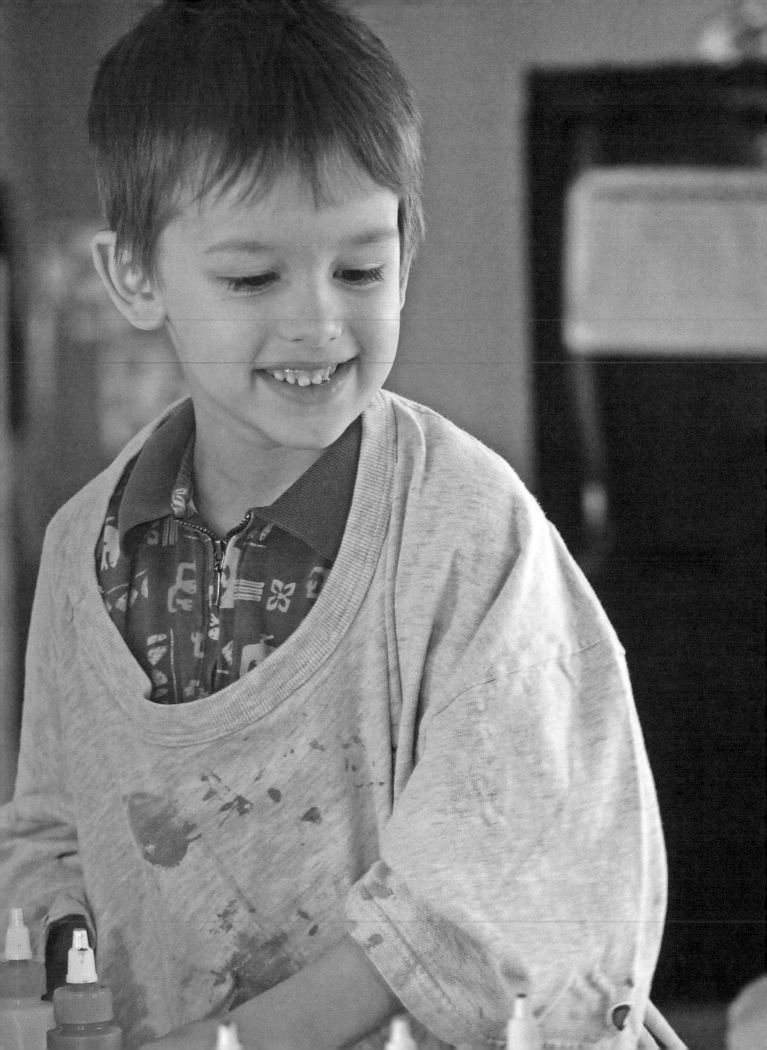

Part 5

<hr/>

Safety and Risk Management

Early care and education programs demonstrate their quality by incorporating a wide variety of process and structural features that address children's needs across all developmental domains. These features are often incorporated into licensing requirements. Child care licensing ensures a minimum level of quality to protect children's safety. Experts agree that this level is very low. It is important for you to consider policies and practices that go beyond licensing requirements. You can enhance the quality of your program and the safety of the care and education children receive.

Children frequently injure themselves in trips and falls, collisions with objects, and scuffles with other children. They are hurt by thrown objects, defective equipment, and more. The Centers for Disease Control and Prevention's Childhood Injury Report (2008) documents unintentional injuries as a common cause of child mortality in the United States. The leading causes of death by unintentional injury differ by age group. For children less than a year old, two-thirds of injury deaths were from suffocation. Drowning was the leading cause of injury death for one- to four-year-olds. For children five to nineteen years old, the most common injury deaths were the result of being occupants in vehicle crashes (Borse et al. 2008).

Although child care environments are usually designed to keep children safe, injuries in child care programs do happen. The Consumer Product Safety Commission (1999) reports that in one year alone, over 31,000 children four years old and younger were treated in U.S. emergency rooms for injuries in child care or school settings. Most injuries in child care programs are minor. But research shows that children who receive minor injuries are at increased risk for additional injuries. They are also more likely to receive severe injuries.

Some unintentional childhood injuries are almost impossible to prevent. Young children are developing coordination and muscle control. Trips and falls with no avoidable cause are very common. Nevertheless, some injuries, especially very severe ones, are preventable. For example, you can prevent many injuries by properly maintaining equipment and surfaces.

You can also prevent injuries and protect children by preparing for natural disasters and emergencies. Fortunately, these are uncommon, but considering the possible disastrous results of these events, you should always be prepared. You may live in an earthquake zone. Your area may experience tornadoes or hurricanes. Emergencies may differ, but many of the preparations are the same. For example, you need to have emergency supplies on hand. You need to be trained to evacuate your facility and to shelter in your facility. You need to know where to get information about emergency events and directions to keep the children safe. You also need to teach the children safety steps so they feel prepared for emergencies as their age and abilities allow.

Some injuries to children are intentionally inflicted, and some of these are severe enough to kill children. **Child abuse** injuries include physical abuse, emotional abuse, sexual abuse, and child neglect. As an early childhood professional, you can do a lot to prevent these injuries and deaths. The Center for the Study of Social Policy (2007) reports that early childhood programs are a powerful force in abuse prevention:

> The uniquely close relationship between caregiver/teacher and parents of young children, the daily opportunities for observation and learning with parents, the relationship between early childhood programs and other resources for parents of young children, and the fact that parents interact with these programs as "empowered consumers" rather than as clients or recipients of a service make this focus a promising universal strategy. (1-1)

Sudden death remains a looming threat to the youngest of children. Over four thousand children die unexpectedly each year. Many of these deaths are unintentional. Some have no apparent cause, even after thorough investigation. Although the causes of some infant deaths cannot be determined, proven strategies can minimize the risks to infants in your care. Changes in infant sleep positions, cribs, crib toys and bedding, and other promising practices are effective in decreasing mortality.

Section 18

Safety

One of the many reasons families use child care programs is to keep their children safe while they are working, studying, or otherwise unavailable. They count on you to protect their children from risks. Young children are just developing their physical and decision-making abilities. They need adults to supervise them and organize their environment to minimize unnecessary risks. Children rely on you to keep indoor and outdoor spaces safe for them to explore. You should select equipment and furnishings that are safe and that stand up to vigorous play. You should use policies and practices that protect children from unnecessary risks.

Safety is also an important part of children's overall well-being and development. It provides a foundation upon which children can grow and flourish. They must feel safe before they can learn and test new skills. A safe environment gives them the confidence to try new things, take appropriate risks, and explore materials and relationships.

Licensing requirements for equipment, water play, pets, transportation, and other safety measures vary a lot. These regulations should be considered the minimum you provide. To truly provide high-quality care and to enhance children's development, you should use best safety practices. These may exceed what is required by your regulatory agencies.

The checklists that follow will help you identify best practices that contribute to high quality. Some of these practices may already be included in your licensing requirements, and others may be new to your program. When an item on a checklist conflicts with your licensing regulations, remember, you *must* comply with the minimum specified in your licensing regulation. If the licensing regulation is less stringent than the recommendation in the checklist, you can also comply with the checklist item, therefore exceeding your licensing regulations.

This section will address:

- Supervising children: Many structural features, such as your room arrangement, contribute to your ability to supervise children. Process features, such as your practices in taking attendance, also contribute to your ability to supervise children.

- Outdoor environment and playground safety: Special attention should be paid to outdoor equipment, maintenance, and supervision practices.

- Indoor environment: Children spend much of their day indoors, and child care spaces require thoughtful planning, selection of safe materials, and maintenance to be safe.

- Transporting children: Transporting children is a huge responsibility requiring special precautions to ensure safety.

- Off-site activities: Activities away from the program's typical space can be very meaningful for children. They also require a lot of planning and attention to supervision.

- Water activities: Water activities present a great opportunity for sensory exploration and fun. They also come with special challenges that merit careful planning and close supervision.

- Animals in the program: Many programs have special pets to help children learn about nature and responsibility. Some precautions are needed to ensure that the animals and children remain safe and healthy.

- Safety education: Children are beginning to explore their world. They need to learn safe ways to navigate the environment.

Supervising Children

Supervising children is an active process. You need to do more than simply observe. You must become involved with children, anticipate what will happen next, and intervene to prevent injuries or harmful incidents.

The environment should be organized to make supervision easy. Regulatory and licensing agencies establish adult-to-child **ratios** to support supervision in child care environments. The ratios state the maximum number of children that can be cared for by one adult. Some states supplement their ratios by requiring adults who supervise groups of children without help from another adult to have certain qualifications. Programs must meet the ratios required by their regulatory agency. To improve the level of supervision, some programs lower ratios so fewer children are cared for by one adult. For example, the licensing requirements may state that four infants can be cared for by one adult, but the program may use the ratio of three infants per adult.

Group sizes are often specified by regulatory agencies. Maximum group sizes are the largest number of children that can be cared for together by any number of adults. For example, a licensing agency may specify the maximum group size of twenty for a group of preschoolers. Only twenty preschoolers can be cared for in one group, no matter how many adults are present.

ENVIRONMENTAL FACTORS

Goal: We plan the environment to optimize supervision of children in our care.

❑ The environment is arranged so children are always visible.

❑ If our setting has small spaces, closets, or other hard-to-supervise spaces, mirrors are used to help with visual supervision.

❑ If infants are cared for, then cribs are kept near the play space. Cribs are not in separate rooms that are unsupervised.

❑ Infant monitors or other mechanical devices are never used to supervise children, even sleeping children.

SUPERVISION PRACTICES

Goal: We use best practices for vigilant supervision of the children in our care.

❑ We care for children using the maximum group sizes and ratios of adults to children recommended by the National Association for the Education of Young Children (NAEYC) in its accreditation standards. (See appendix H for NAEYC's Accreditation Standards Teacher-Child Ratios within Group Sizes.)

❑ Each child's arrival at the program is recorded each day.

❑ Attendance is taken many times each day to ensure that each child is present and is being supervised.

❑ The children are counted, and attendance is taken every time they move between spaces: indoors to outdoors, room to room, and outdoors to indoors. Names and faces are matched to each class list.

❑ Groups of children are constantly supervised. The required adult-to-child ratio is maintained, even when adults take a break, retrieve supplies, or make phone calls.

❑ Children are properly supervised when their needs differ from the rest of the group's. For example, if a child needs to use the toilet while others are on the playground, that child is supervised.

❑ Daily activities are planned so children are properly supervised during **transitions**, especially when families are arriving and departing.

❑ Breaks and lunchtimes for teachers are planned so children are supervised during naps.

❑ Teachers are physically present in the room with children, even during naptime.

❑ Teachers work as a team to supervise indoor and outdoor spaces.

Did you know? If you are lucky enough to have colleagues supervising with you, be sure you spread out in the space. Each teacher should be responsible for some of the space. Adults are tempted to cluster together and talk while children are busy playing. But children need your attention 100 percent of the time. If you and your colleagues are close enough to easily carry on a conversation using your indoor voices, you are too close and probably not supervising your space responsibly.

❑ Teachers position themselves on the playground so that they can observe and interact with all children.

❑ Teachers routinely move around all areas where children are present to supervise them closely.

❑ Teachers position themselves so they can see as much of the space as possible. For example, they sit with their backs to a corner so they can scan the entire room or playground.

❑ Teachers are trained to supervise children indoors and outdoors.

Outdoor Environment and Playground Safety

Outdoor play is an essential part of any early childhood program. During outdoor play, children use their muscles and are physically active. Vigorous play is good for their health and overall development. Most important, children really enjoy the outdoors.

The outdoor spaces used by early childhood programs vary. Some programs have very elaborate, commercially designed playgrounds and play equipment. Others have residential or home-made equipment. Still others have natural playscapes. All types of playgrounds and playground equipment are potentially safe for use by children, but equipment must meet the standards of the U.S. Consumer Product Safety Commission (CPSC) and ASTM International.

You can determine if your program's playground meets these standards by having a Certified Playground Safety Inspector (CPSI) inspect the playground and its equipment. You can locate a certified inspector by visiting one of these two websites:

National Recreation and Park Association (NRPA) https://ipv.nrpa.org/CPSI_registry/

National Program for Playground Safety www.playgroundsafety.org

Outdoor play equipment must be placed on shock-absorbing materials or surfaces to prevent injuries from falls. **Use zones** are the spaces beneath and extending at least six feet in all directions beyond the area where outdoor equipment is located. These zones must be constantly maintained to be effective. For example, mulch must be raked so its depth remains consistent in high-traffic areas. Remember that ice and snow in cold weather areas can make shock-absorbing materials less effective in protecting children when they fall. You may need to close some areas of the playground when ice forms in use zones.

Safe equipment and surfaces are only one part of playground safety. Supervision and safe play practices are equally important. Young children are just learning how to use their emerging physical abilities. Your supervision and interactions help them make wise choices and play safely.

OUTDOOR ENVIRONMENT AND PLAYGROUND SAFETY

Goal: We protect children's safety by keeping children's well-being in mind when designing and using our outdoor play spaces.

❑ The program's adult-to-child ratios and group sizes are maintained during outdoor play.

❑ The playground space contains at least 75 square feet for each child using it at one time. For example, if twenty children use the playground together, they need 1,500 square feet.

❑ The program supervises the entire outdoor area using a team approach. Adults move around the play area, scanning the space and avoiding distractions, such as conversations with other adults.

❑ Adults interact with the children during outdoor play in ways that permit careful supervision.

❑ A first aid kit is available on the playground so staff members can give minor first aid without leaving the area.

❑ The program practices routine maintenance of the playground, including equipment, use zones, and landscaping.

❑ Separate outdoor spaces with age-appropriate equipment are available and used by infants, toddlers, preschoolers, and school-age children.

❑ School-age children do not use the same playground space at the same time as younger children.

❑ Play areas do not include trampolines or ball pits.

Did you know? Full-sized and mini trampolines are not recommended for children under six years of age. *Caring for Our Children: National Health and Safety Standards* states, "The trampoline has no place in outdoor playgrounds and should never be regarded as play equipment" (AAP et al. 2011, 276). Many activities can substitute for trampolines. For example, jump roping is a safer way for children to practice jumping and get aerobic **exercise**.

❏ Shaded areas are available for children's use and cover at least 30 percent of the play area.

❏ Sand play areas are covered when not in use and are effectively drained.

❏ The playground is monitored for standing water. If it is found, steps are taken to drain it.

❏ Landscaping and plants on the playground or within reach of children are not poisonous.

Did you know? If you don't know if the plants in your landscaping are poisonous, take samples to a local garden store, horticultural society, or agricultural extension office for advice. If you know the names of the plants, you can check online resources for lists of nonpoisonous and poisonous plants.

❏ Bike helmets are required when children use bicycles, tricycles, and scooters.

❏ Children are not permitted to wear necklaces, hoods with strings, or other dangling items while using playground equipment.

❏ Sidewalks are routinely swept to prevent slips, trips, and falls from loose sand or gravel.

❏ The outdoor space is inspected each day before children use it. Debris, litter, and other materials that can cause injury are removed.

❏ Our program purchases new outdoor equipment to ensure access to recall information, damage history (if any), and relevant warranties.

❏ The outdoor equipment is inspected each day to identify wear and tear. Equipment that has developed cracks, splinters, rust, corrosion, holes, chipped paint, exposed anchors, or other hazards is removed until repaired or disposed of.

❏ Accidents on the playground, even minor ones, are documented. Staff members routinely review the records to look for trends and to enhance the safety of space, equipment, and practices.

Did you know? The U.S. Consumer Product Safety Commission publishes an excellent handbook on making your playground a safe and engaging outdoor play space. *The Public Playground Safety Handbook* (2010) is available online at www.cpsc.gov/cpscpub/pubs/325.pdf.

Bonus Checklist

❑ The playground and equipment have been inspected by a certified inspector. They meet the CPSC and ASTM international standards. If anything was deemed substandard, children can no longer use it, and plans for repair or replacement are in place.

Indoor Environment

Spaces used by early childhood programs vary widely. High-quality programs are found in residential homes, commercial spaces, churches, schools, and public buildings. All spaces must meet some requirements to minimize risks to children.

The indoor environment includes the facility itself and the toys, equipment, and decorations used to enrich it. Licensing regulations often include specific rules for the space where children receive care. They may have fewer rules about the furnishings and equipment used there.

The U.S. Consumer Product Safety Commission (CPSC) is responsible for testing toys and other materials for children to determine their safety. The CPSC routinely issues recalls of materials determined to be unsafe for children's use. You can register to receive e-mail notices of these recalls by visiting the CPSC website at www.cpsc.gov.

Programs providing infant care require specialized equipment, including cribs. Cribs are the best place for infants to sleep. They are safer than swings, car seats, bassinets, and other places where infants may fall asleep. But not all cribs are as safe as they should be. In fact, more infants die in incidents involving cribs than any other piece of nursery equipment. Most incidents involve older cribs manufactured before stringent standards for crib safety were established.

In 2010, the U.S. Consumer Product Safety Act developed safety standards for full-sized and non-full-sized cribs. These standards ended the sales of drop-side cribs. They also ordered stronger mattress supports and crib hardware and made safety testing of cribs more rigorous. As of June 2011, cribs that did not meet the new standards could no longer be manufactured. Most important for child care programs, starting in December 2012 centers and family child care homes can no longer use cribs that do not comply with the enhanced standards. The enhanced standards eliminate the use of most cribs with sides that drop (CPSC 2011). While this change can be costly, it can also prevent injuries and save lives. Compliance is critical.

INDOOR SPACE AND MATERIALS

Goal: Our indoor spaces and materials are selected and maintained to protect children's safety.

❏ The indoor space used by children contains at least thirty-five square feet for each child in care.

❏ We document the facility's compliance with all fire codes, sanitation requirements, and health codes.

❏ All of the toys and materials in the environment meet the U.S. Consumer Products Safety Commission standards.

❏ Small objects, toys, or toy parts are not accessible to children under three years of age. Toys or objects with removable parts less than 1¼ inches in diameter are potential choking hazards.

Did you know? Young children put anything and everything in their mouths. Rather than estimating what materials are safe or unsafe, best practice is to measure questionable items using a choke tube. Choke tubes can be purchased where childhood safety supplies are sold or from most early childhood vendors.

❏ Plastic bags, small round objects (smaller than 1¾ inches in diameter), sharp objects (such as pins, staples, or tacks), magnets, marbles, safety pins, and Styrofoam objects are not accessible to children under three years of age.

❏ The indoor environment and materials are inspected each day to identify wear and tear. Anything that has developed sharp corners, chipped paint, holes, tears, rough edges, loose buttons, or other hazards is removed from children's use. It is either repaired or disposed of.

❏ Our floors are level, and carpets and rugs have nonskid, low-nap surfaces to minimize trips and falls.

❏ Shelves, bookcases, and other heavy equipment are securely fixed in place so children can't pull them over, become trapped behind them, pinch their limbs, or become injured during earthquakes.

❏ Water tables and trays are drained, cleaned, and sanitized at least daily.

❏ Water tables and trays are covered when not in use.

❑ Cords from electrical devices, window blinds, or other sources are secured out of reach of the children, including those in cribs.

❑ Latex balloons are not permitted in the children's environment.

Did you know? Balloons seem like innocent toys. They fascinate young children. But balloons, especially latex balloons, also present hazards. Young children may be allergic to latex, which can cause potentially dangerous reactions. When balloons break, as they all eventually do, their pieces become choking hazards. Soft balls are better choices for throwing and catching.

❑ Indoor plants are nonpoisonous.

❑ Securely installed gates or other guards are located at the top and bottom of stairs in the children's space. Security gates have latching devices that can be easily operated only by adults. No pressure gates or accordion gates are used.

❑ Stairs used by children are equipped with securely installed handrails at children's height.

❑ Doors in the children's space have covered hinges to prevent pinched fingers or toes.

❑ Windows cannot be opened unless screens are securely in place and safety barriers are installed.

❑ Fans are not placed within reach of children, including children in cribs or on changing tables.

❑ Rolling walkers, umbrella strollers, accordion gates, playpens, portable cribs, and vinyl tents are never used.

❑ Teachers' purses and bags are locked away to prevent children from accessing the contents.

❑ Diaper bags or backpacks are either kept out of reach or checked daily to be sure no hazards such as diaper cream or medication are accessible.

❑ Our program uses only covered, hands-free trash cans. When they are full, the trash is removed from the facility.

❑ Our program has a recycling program, and adults model recycling practices for the children.

Did you know? The U.S. Consumer Product Safety Commission publishes an excellent resource on selecting toys and equipment for your program. *For Kids' Sake: Think Toy Safety* is available online at www.cpsc.gov/cpscpub/pubs/281.pdf. Consider sharing this resource with families in your program.

CRIBS

If you do not care for infants and don't use cribs, continue to the next checklist, Transporting Children.

Goal: Infants are safe while sleeping in our care.

❑ Cribs meet the 2011 Consumer Product Safety Commission standards.

Did you know? The recent changes to crib standards represent a significant change for many programs. You should thoroughly investigate the new standards and compare them to the cribs you are using in your program. More information about crib standards can be found on the CPSC's Crib Information Center, www.cpsc.gov/info/cribs/index.html.

❑ Cribs, including crib mattresses, are checked regularly, at least weekly, for signs of wear and tear, such as cracks, tears, splinters, or loose screws or nuts.

❑ Cribs are cleaned and sanitized weekly.

❑ Cribs are never modified or adjusted from the original manufacturer's recommendations.

❑ At least one crib for each four children in care is reinforced so that it can be used for **evacuation** of infants from the facility.

Transporting Children

The responsibility for transporting children should not be taken lightly. Motor vehicle crashes are the most common cause of death among children ages three to fourteen years. To be as safe as possible while riding in vehicles, children should be seated securely in child **vehicle safety restraints** of the right size and type for their age and size. The proper use of vehicle safety restraints (car seats and booster seats) can dramatically decrease the risks to young children during transport. But to be effective, the restraints must fit the vehicle properly, be installed properly, and fit the children who are using them properly.

Besides using appropriate vehicle safety restraints, you must pay attention to vehicle maintenance, safety procedures, supervision, and safe driving. Driving a vehicle requires concentration and skill. Supervising children while operating a vehicle is challenging. You should consider your driving record and your level of comfort and experience as a driver before deciding to transport children. Review your licensing regulations on transporting children. They may specify who can provide transportation, the types of vehicles that can be used, and the minimum safety practices required.

TRANSPORTING CHILDREN

Goal: Children in our program are transported safely.

❑ Children are transported only with specific, written consent from their families.

❑ The program's adult-to-child ratios are maintained while children are being transported. The driver of the vehicle is not counted in the ratio.

❑ Children are always supervised when in vehicles. Adult-to-child ratios are maintained at all times, even while waiting to depart.

❑ The appropriate vehicle safety restraint (car seat or booster seat) is used, based on each child's age, weight, and height.

❑ All adults who install vehicle safety restraints in vehicles or who buckle children into vehicle safety restraints have been trained by the program's child care health consultant or someone designated by our regulatory agency.

❑ Vehicle safety restraints are always used according to the manufacturer's instructions.

❑ Vehicle safety restraints are in good repair and show no evidence of having been in a vehicle accident.

❑ Metal parts of vehicle safety restraints are checked to be sure they are not hot before children are placed in the seat.

❑ Children under age thirteen are not permitted to ride in the front seat of any vehicle.

❑ Drivers responsible for transporting children are at least twenty-one years of age and possess the appropriate license for the vehicle.

❑ Drivers have a documented safe driving record, no criminal records of crimes against children, and are routinely drug tested.

❑ Before transporting children, drivers are trained to use vehicle safety restraints, car seats, booster seats, seat belts, and emergency procedures.

❑ Drivers are certified in first aid and pediatric **cardiopulmonary resuscitation** (CPR).

❑ Program-owned vehicles and vehicles used by the program are supplied with emergency equipment, including a first aid kit, flashlight, and **fire extinguisher**.

❏ Staff members bring along emergency information and emergency supplies for each child in the vehicle.

❏ Staff members have a way to summon help, such as a cell phone, when transporting children.

❏ Children are only transported when the route to and from the destination is well known. The driver is familiar with emergency resources and routes to emergency care resources in the area.

❏ A plan is in place for parking the vehicle and for loading and unloading the children in a safe area.

❏ Children are never allowed to stand or lie down while being transported.

❏ Before and during the trip, teachers talk with the children about safe transportation behavior such as staying seated and wearing seat belts.

❏ Smoking in or around the vehicle is prohibited, even when children are not in the vehicle.

❏ Staff members do not plan trips that require children to be in a vehicle for over an hour at a time.

❏ The temperature of the vehicle is checked before children are loaded in the vehicle and then routinely during the trip. Vehicles should be air-conditioned if over 82 degrees Fahrenheit, and heated if cooler than 65 degrees Fahrenheit.

❏ Staff members take attendance, checking children's names and faces as children board and leave the vehicle.

❏ Each adult (staff members and volunteers) in the vehicle knows the number of children aboard.

❏ During the trip, all adults in the vehicle avoid distracting the driver of the vehicle. They also avoid behaviors that distract from the supervision of the children. For example, they do not talk on cell phones, send text or e-mail messages, wear earphones, or eat.

❏ Staff members check the entire vehicle after unloading to be sure that all children have left the vehicle.

❑ Program-owned vehicles are maintained according to the manufacturer's recommendations, including preventive maintenance. Records are kept of routine maintenance.

❑ The interiors of program-owned vehicles are cleaned at the end of each day the vehicle has been used.

❑ Staff members check the vehicle before each trip for broken seats, cracked windows, frayed belts, or other safety hazards. These inspections are documented.

❑ The program keeps written records of the vehicle's insurance, maintenance, and drivers' qualifications and training, including their license numbers.

Did you know? When planning off-site trips or transporting children, you may need to consider their medications. Are medications needed while you're away from the facility? If so, consider what will be needed to safely store, transport, and administer them. Sometimes it's possible to change the schedule for a child's medication to avoid giving it while you're away from the facility. This requires careful coordination with the child's family, and possibly the physician, so advanced planning is essential.

Bonus Checklist

❑ Our program partners with community safety professionals to offer car seat safety checks to families on a regular basis.

Off-Site Activities

Off-site activities, such as field trips and neighborhood walks, can enhance your program for young children. Visiting places and people in the community exposes children to new ideas and activities that you can't replicate in your program. For some children, off-site activities or field trips may be their only chances to experience some of the rich learning opportunities your community offers.

When you leave the facility with young children, you accept new challenges to ensuring the children's health and safety. Away from your program, some things are out of your complete control. Therefore, the decision to leave your program's facility can never be a light one.

Off-site activities require advanced planning and a high level of supervision. Excursions often involve transporting children, so be aware of the considerations described in Transporting Children. Before any trip, consider the merits of the activity. Think carefully about the destination's appropriateness for the ages and abilities of the children in your group. Is the activity something the children will enjoy? Will they understand and participate in it fully? Could you replicate it in your facility? Does the trip add something special to your program that cannot be accomplished in another way? Off-site activities require a lot of time and effort. They come with some risks. Be certain the benefits are well worth your efforts.

OFF-SITE ACTIVITIES

Goal: Children are safely supervised during off-site activities.

❑ Children are taken on walks or trips away from the facility only with written permission from their families specific to each trip.

❑ A staff member visits the destination before the children's trip to check for safety hazards and to become familiar with amenities like restrooms, drinking fountains, and emergency resources.

❑ The program's adult-to-child ratio is maintained on trips. At least one additional adult is present throughout the trip.

❑ Teachers take attendance regularly, counting each child and matching the child's name and face to the group list.

❑ Teachers carry emergency information for each child on the trip.

❑ Each child on the trip wears a wristlet, T-shirt, or button identifying the child as a member of the group, including contact information for the program.

❑ During off-site activities, children's first or last names are never visible on their shirts, jackets, backpacks, or other wear.

❑ Off-site playgrounds are inspected by staff members before children use the equipment.

❑ Teachers carry first aid supplies, including those for treating allergic reactions, even if it is likely that supplies are available at the destination.

❑ Substitutes, temporary employees, student workers, or volunteers are never used to meet the adult-to-child ratio for off-site trips.

❏ Teachers carry cell phones so they can summon help or communicate with staff members at the facility.

❏ Children are directly supervised by teachers at all times on trips, including during activities. For example, teachers sit with children at movies or plays and accompany children to restrooms.

Did you know? Before leaving for an off-site activity, prepare the children for what will happen and what behavior will be expected. Talk with the children about where you will be going, what kinds of activities you will do there, and what the place will be like. If possible, show pictures from previous trips to this destination. Discuss any special rules for children's behavior during the trip or during transport to the destination. For example, if you expect children to be quiet during a movie or a play, demonstrate and practice the behavior you expect. Give children a chance to ask questions and to express their concerns about the plans. Preparing children in advance helps them have smooth transitions and increases everyone's enjoyment.

Water Activities

Children love playing in water. Water play can also be an important learning activity. When children pour, scoop, splash, and swirl water, they learn about cause and effect, weights and measures, and the physical properties of things. Water play can range from using small tubs and trays to swimming pools. No matter the size of the water container or pool, you need to exercise caution. Children should not be exposed to illness and infection, insects, or drowning.

Many regulatory agencies specify lower than usual adult-child ratios for water activities and swimming. They may also require the presence of someone certified as a **lifeguard** when children are in or near a swimming pool. The American Red Cross offers a comprehensive program for certifying lifeguards. This special training is essential when you are supervising swimming pools and swimming activities. You may be a very accomplished swimmer and comfortable in the water supervising young children, but these are not acceptable substitutes for the presence of a certified lifeguard.

Swimming pools and hot tubs are treated chemically to kill germs and prevent the spread of illness and infection. These chemicals help protect the health of swimmers, but they also pose a threat if they are not handled properly. Children should never have access to pool chemicals.

Swimming pools, wading pools, hot tubs, even large buckets of water can be hazardous—even when they are not being used. Children can easily fall into water and become endangered with just a momentary lapse of supervision. Even one inch of standing water can prove to be a safety hazard. This is why most pools and hot tubs must be securely fenced. Anytime children are near water, they must be closely supervised by sight, sound, and touch (they should be within your reach).

WATER TABLES, TUBS, AND SPRINKLERS

Goal: Children in our program engage in water play that is well supervised and safe.

❑ Teachers closely supervise children when they are engaged in water play.

❑ Teachers ensure that children do not drink water from water play containers.

❑ Water play toys are sanitized each day.

❑ Sprinklers are moved regularly to prevent puddles and slippery grass.

❑ Teachers supervising water play are trained in first aid and CPR.

Did you know? Squirt bottles can be fun, and very safe, water play alternatives for warm days. Children enjoy squirting spray bottles and the cooling mist they produce. During squirt bottle play, avoid spraying water directly into children's faces and discourage them from spraying one another in the face.

POOLS

Goal: Children in our program use wading or swimming pools that are well supervised and safe.

❑ The program maintains enhanced adult-to-child ratios during wading or swimming pool use: infants, 1:1; toddlers, 1:1; preschoolers, 1:4; and school-age children, 1:6.

❑ A certified lifeguard is on duty when children use a swimming pool. The lifeguard is not included in the adult-to-child ratio.

❑ Swimming pools meet all of the standards set by the health department, including those for warning signs and safety equipment. Pools are regularly inspected.

Did you know? Safety requirements for swimming pools are regularly updated. For example, requirements for pool drain covers have recently been updated in many areas. If your program has a pool on site, you are responsible for staying abreast of changes in pool regulations.

❑ If the program has a swimming pool, it is fenced to prevent unsupervised access by children.

❑ If the program has a swimming pool, pool chemicals and equipment are stored in a locked storage area inaccessible to children.

❑ Children are never allowed in or near hot tubs, saunas, whirlpool tubs, or spas.

❑ Water temperature for swimming pools is maintained at 82 to 88 degrees Fahrenheit when the pool is in use.

❑ Staff members routinely check to be sure that swimming children are not cold or overheated.

❑ Each child's swimming ability and comfort in the water are evaluated and discussed with the child's family before children are allowed in a pool.

❑ Approved flotation devices (life jackets) are available and are fitted to children who require them. Inflatable arm bands (water wings) are not used.

❑ Floating toys like air mattresses or inflatable rings are never allowed in pools.

❑ The program does not use portable wading pools.

Did you know? Sprinklers, spray bottles, and hoses are safer and healthier alternatives to wading pools. Water in wading pools is not filtered or treated, so it is impossible to provide adequate sanitation, especially for very young children, who may not yet be fully toilet trained.

Animals in the Program

Caring for animals offers learning opportunities to young children. Besides learning about animals, children can also learn **empathy** and responsibility when they are involved in pet care. Keeping animals in your program also requires your time and attention, because young children can rarely perform the tasks needed to maintain animals' health.

Some animals are better choices for interacting with young children than others. Furry animals may present problems for children with respiratory problems or children allergic to dander. Some animals like turtles may carry **salmonella**, which can be transmitted to the children. Such animals (usually reptiles and amphibians) are not good choices for your program.

Once your program has decided to care for a pet, you need to put precautions in place to ensure the health of the pet and of the children. Animals require feeding and clean surroundings. They also require medical care and maintenance, such as nail trimming and grooming. Care requires your time and commitment and can be expensive. Carefully consider all aspects of pet care before committing to an animal.

Any staff member in your program who is pregnant must take additional precautions around cat litter boxes. Litter boxes should be cleaned daily but not by pregnant women, who can acquire the infection toxoplasmosis from infected cat waste. Even cats that appear to be healthy may transmit this infection from their feces.

ANIMALS IN THE PROGRAM

Goal: Our selection of and care for animals protects children's health and safety.

❑ We have no animals in the program that are likely to transmit salmonella: lizards, snakes, iguanas, ferrets, birds of the parrot family, or turtles.

❑ All animals are in good health and are fully immunized.

❑ Health records from a veterinarian are on file for each animal.

❑ Stray animals have not been adopted by the program.

❑ Teachers instruct children about caring for animals and appropriate ways to interact with them.

❑ Teachers wash hands and supervise the children in washing hands before and after touching animals and their cages, food, or supplies.

❑ Staff members wear gloves when cleaning animals, their cages or bedding, or fish aquariums.

❑ Teachers supervise closely when children interact with animals. We remain close enough to step in immediately if the child or the animal shows distress.

❑ The program's animals are never permitted in food preparation or food service areas.

❑ Animal food and supplies are kept out of children's reach.

❑ Animal cages and bedding are kept clean and in good repair.

❑ Children are not allowed to touch animal waste, including litter boxes, mulch, or straw.

❑ Children are not permitted to kiss or touch animals with their mouths.

Did you know? Sometimes children try to show their affection for pets by snuggling them to their faces or even kissing them. You should discourage children from hugging pets too tightly and kissing them, even on their fur. Instead, suggest that children blow a kiss to the animal or use gentle petting to show their affection. Demonstrating gentle petting helps children understand how to interact with animals.

❑ Families are notified about program animals when they enroll.

❑ Staff members are trained in feeding, cleaning, and exposing animals to extreme temperatures.

Did you know? Selecting a pet for children in the program requires research and planning. Younger children may be better suited to fish or other pets they can watch but can't touch. Older children may value the chance to hold, pet, and help care for an animal like a rabbit or gerbil. Before you commit to any pet, talk with the children and the families so you fully understand their level of interest and commitment to a pet. You'll also learn about potential challenges like allergies. The children may enjoy helping you to do some research about pets. Many excellent children's books can be used to help you explain pet care and the responsibilities that come with pet ownership. Consult a professional, like a veterinarian, to be sure you are selecting a pet that is a good match for groups of young children.

Safety Education

Sometimes children overestimate what they can do. When they first acquire new skills, they feel powerful and are eager to try out their new abilities. They may not realize their abilities need practice to become expert. Think of children learning to ride a scooter. Once they have the basic movements down, they may still need to perfect balance and coordination to go fast or maneuver around obstacles. These skills come with time, practice, and support from you.

Sometimes children underestimate the risks associated with behaviors adults or older children engage in. For example, young children may see older children climb to the top of playground equipment and assume they can do the same. But their emerging skills may not yet be up to the task. Their learning often involves falls or injuries, such as scraped knees.

While children are learning about their abilities and the risks around them, they need support from you. You are responsible for protecting them from potential serious injury. You supervise and organize a safe environment for them. You can also help children remain safe by teaching them how to protect themselves. Learning safe practices benefits children throughout their lives.

SAFETY EDUCATION

Goal: We plan and implement activities to help children learn about safety.

❑ Teachers plan lessons and activities that reinforce safe habits, such as hygiene, safe play, and personal safety.

❑ Teachers use incidents to teach children about choices and consequences.

❑ Teachers use special events, such as a visit by a firefighter or a field trip to a fire station, to discuss safety topics.

❑ Our program uses community resources, such as firefighters, police officers, and health care professionals, to teach children about safety.

❑ Our program gives families information to reinforce safety lessons at home.

Did you know? One great way to help children learn basic safety lessons is children's literature. Many children's books describe learning to ride a bicycle, playing at the playground, interacting with pets, and other safety topics. Your local bookseller or children's librarian can help you find books on topics that fit the needs of the children in your care.

Section 19

Emergency Preparedness

Despite your best efforts to keep children healthy and safe, emergencies happen. Some emergencies cannot be predicted, such as earthquakes. Others, such as storms and tornadoes, can sometimes be anticipated but not prevented. In all cases, thoughtful planning and preparation can minimize the dangers of emergencies. Different geographic areas have unique risks, so you should contact your licensing agency or emergency management agency to understand the local risks and resources. Excellent resources for emergency planning can be found in the *Head Start Emergency Preparedness Manual.* You can download this manual from the U.S. Department of Health and Human Services Early Learning Knowledge Center at http://eclkc.ohs.acf.hhs.gov /hslc/tta-system/health/ep/Head_Start_Emergency_Preparedness_Manual.pdf.

Some planning and preparation for emergencies require children's involvement. For example, children must participate in fire drills so they are prepared if a fire occurs. When you involve children in drills or other emergency preparations, do not unnecessarily alarm them. Children should feel safe and confident in your program. Take time to explain carefully what will be happening and why the preparations are needed. Invite the children to talk about their experiences and feelings after the preparedness activities. Allow them to express their emotions and have their questions answered. For example, during fire safety month, you can talk about fire drills and why your program has these drills. Tell them it is very unlikely that a fire will happen, but that you still practice so that you can be extremely safe. You can also tell them that the practice will be exciting, maybe even fun, but also very important. If possible, allow children to hear the sound of the fire alarm so they know exactly what to expect. Apply these techniques to other preparedness activities, such as sheltering drills (tornado drills) or earthquake drills.

This section will address:

- General emergency preparedness: Some emergency procedures are helpful in almost any situation. This checklist addresses emergency contact information, emergency supplies, and other all-purpose emergency procedures.

- Fire safety: Fires, although rare, are extremely dangerous. These precautions help prevent fires and address preparedness when fires occur.

- Severe weather safety: Weather can be unpredictable. Sometimes it poses dangers to children. Although weather events cannot be prevented, your program can prepare to minimize danger to children.

- Earthquake safety: Some areas are susceptible to the hazards associated with earthquakes. Like weather emergencies, earthquakes cannot be prevented. Precautions can minimize damage and injuries.

- Medical emergency preparedness: Most injuries to children are minor. Sometimes, despite all of your precautions, children unexpectedly require the attention of medical professionals.

General Emergency Preparedness

Some elements of emergencies can be anticipated and prepared for. For example, you may need to evacuate your facility. Preparing for and practicing an **evacuation** promote safety when an emergency occurs. Other emergency situations require unique preparations.

GENERAL EMERGENCY PREPAREDNESS

Goal: We protect children from dangers that cannot be prevented.

❑ Our program's child care health consultant has reviewed and approved all of our emergency procedures.

❑ Our facility's street numbers are clearly posted on the facility's exterior and are visible from the street.

❑ Emergency phone numbers for fire, police, and poison control are posted by each telephone.

❑ A working telephone is in each space used by the children.

❑ Battery-powered flashlights are present in each area used by the children, including vehicles, restrooms, and nap areas.

❑ Emergency contact information for each child is on file in the space where children receive care.

❑ Emergency contact information is available on a mobile device or is secured in an off-site location so it can be used in the event of an evacuation.

❑ At least two emergency exits lead directly to a ground-level outdoor area.

❑ Each exit from our facility is clear, indoors and outdoors, from furniture, supplies, trash, or other obstacles. No outdoor buildup of ice or snow blocks children's safe and speedy exit.

❑ Maps illustrating primary and secondary **evacuation routes** are easy to understand and are posted in each child care space.

❑ At least one infant crib designed for evacuation is available for every four infants enrolled in our program.

❑ All staff members are familiar with our plan for what each adult should do if evacuation occurs.

❑ At least one first aid kit is present in each space where children receive care. These include outdoor areas, vehicles used by children, and areas where children nap and eat.

❑ First aid kits are easily accessible to adults but out of reach of children.

❑ Two days of supplies such as food, water, and diapers are on hand for use in emergencies or disasters when assistance may not be available for extended periods.

❑ Staff members are trained in procedures to **shelter in place** when evacuation is not appropriate.

❑ Two locations are planned for shelter away from the facility. These can be used if children cannot return to the facility after an evacuation. Permission to use the shelter facilities has been obtained.

❑ Families are given information about the shelter locations when they enroll.

❑ The children rehearse evacuating the child care facility at a minimum every thirty days or as required by the licensing agency.

❑ One staff member is designated to communicate with emergency responders during an emergency.

Did you know? In the aftermath of emergencies or disasters, children may struggle to understand what has happened and how their world has changed. Like adults, children may experience fear, grief, and confusion during and after traumatic events. You can help them develop resilience and provide reassurance and comfort in times of great stress. Part 3 of this book addresses emotional health and resilience and provides many helpful ideas. You may also benefit from a booklet written by the late Jim Greenman in the aftermath of Hurricanes Katrina and Rita, *What Happened to My World? Helping Children Cope with Natural Disaster and Catastrophe*. It is available online at www/brighthorizons.com /talktochildren/docs/What_Happened_to_My_World.pdf.

Fire Safety

Although fires in child care programs are rare, they can be devastating. Practice the procedures that minimize the risk of fire, and prepare yourself and the children to act quickly and safely if fire occurs.

Fires can be the result of cooking incidents, electrical problems, or unsafe operation of equipment like space heaters. Regular inspections of your facility are one of the best ways to prevent fires. Inspectors can assess risks from many potential fire sources. They can evaluate the procedures and equipment that alert you of fire and assist you in evacuating the facility safely. Forming partnerships with local fire authorities also gives you another community resource to use in developing safety programs for the children.

Young children are ready to learn and practice basic safety procedures to protect them in emergencies at home and elsewhere. Regularly rehearse evacuations of the facility, including use of reinforced evacuation cribs for infants. During your rehearsals, do not frighten the children unnecessarily. Practice crouching or crawling to avoid smoke.

When children reach preschool age, they are ready to practice the stop, drop, and roll technique used to extinguish clothing fires. Remind the children that they are unlikely to ever need this skill, but that it is always good to practice, just in case. Many online resources support you in planning activities to teach fire safety skills to children. For example, the "Sparky" website (www.sparky.org) has a variety of child-oriented resources, including pages that illustrate the stop, drop, and roll procedure.

FIRE SAFETY

Goal: We protect children from the dangers of a facility fire.

❑ Our facility has been inspected and approved by a fire marshal, fire safety inspector, or another inspector. These inspectors based their inspections on local fire codes and the National Fire Protection Association's Life Safety Code.

❑ Our facility provides fire and smoke detectors in spaces used by children and on each floor of the facility, even those not used by children.

❑ All **fire extinguishers** are labeled *A*, *B*, or *C* and are regularly maintained.

❑ Staff members are trained to use fire extinguishers. They know that their first responsibility is to evacuate the children.

❏ Portable space heaters using unvented gas, oil, or kerosene are not used.

❏ Electric space heaters are used according to manufacturer's instructions. They are never placed within reach of children, are at least three feet from curtains, papers, furniture, and any flammable objects, and are observed while in use.

❏ Fireplaces and wood or corn pellet stoves are inaccessible to children. They are installed in compliance with building codes and are used and maintained according to manufacturers' instructions.

❏ Our program practices fire drills at least once each month. We document the results of the drill, including the time required for complete evacuation and any obstacles to efficient evacuation.

Did you know? When you plan fire drills, be sure to vary not only the days of the week but also the times of day when they occur. While some times of day are inconvenient for drills, such as naptime, arrival, and departure, it is still important to rehearse them during these times because you can't predict when a fire may occur.

❏ A meeting place outside the facility has been designated for use after evacuation.

❏ An indoor space away from the facility has been chosen for use as a waiting area when children cannot return to the facility and the weather is bad.

❏ Teachers carry attendance information and children's emergency information when they evacuate.

❏ Teachers receive training on how to respond to a fire emergency before they begin working with children.

❏ Teachers teach the children fire safety, including safe evacuation of the facility and use of the stop, drop, and roll technique.

Severe Weather Safety

Nothing is more unpredictable than the weather. Most of the time, bad weather is just an inconvenience. Sometimes weather is so severe that it can pose a real threat to you, the children, and their families. The weather-related emergencies that may affect your facility vary by location. For example, some areas are prone to tornadoes, while others experience hurricanes, flooding, or wildfires. Be aware of the potential risks in your own area.

Weather-related emergencies may not require evacuation of your facility. For example, when a hurricane is predicted, authorities may recommend that the facility be evacuated. But during a tornado, evacuation of the facility may be very dangerous. The type of weather, the predicted severity, the timing, and the availability of evacuation sites may all impact when evacuation is the best course of action. Your local emergency management agency can help you plan for different kinds of weather-related emergencies. Listen to National Oceanic and Atmospheric Administration (**NOAA**) announcements to determine your response.

When evacuation is not needed, sheltering in the facility is often the recommended safety strategy. Sheltering is necessary when it is unsafe to evacuate your facility. For example, during a tornado, sheltering children in a basement or interior room in the facility is safer than attempting to evacuate. During severe weather, the best rooms for sheltering in place are interior rooms away from doors, exterior walls, and especially windows. Designated shelter spaces should be on the ground floor. In the case of tornadoes, use the facility's basement if it has one.

SEVERE WEATHER SAFETY

Goal: Our policies and procedures protect children from risks associated with severe weather.

- ❏ Our program keeps a NOAA weather radio in a central location in the facility. It has a tone alert and a backup battery.

- ❏ We have designated shelter spaces where staff members can protect children and ourselves.

- ❏ Our designated shelter spaces are labeled.

- ❏ Our shelter spaces contain emergency supplies, including a first aid kit, flashlight, water, nonperishable food, and a telephone.

Did you know? You should consider stocking shelter spaces with books, games, or other activities that appeal to a broad range of children. If you must wait in the shelter for an extended time, a few activities can help to pass the time and calm restless, possibly scared children.

❑ We have a written process for notifying families if the program must close for weather-related or other emergencies.

❑ We have a written procedure that describes how staff members will escort children to and care for children in designated shelter spaces.

❑ Teachers bring attendance information and children's emergency information to the designated shelter spaces.

❑ Children are not allowed to play outdoors until local authorities have issued an all clear for the area.

❑ Children do not use outdoor play equipment when it is wet or covered in snow.

❑ During weather-related emergency seasons, teachers practice escorting children to designated shelter spaces at least monthly.

❑ Records are kept of our program's weather-related emergency practices.

❑ Our weather-related emergency practice records are reviewed annually with the help of our program's child care health consultant, who looks for ways to improve our practices.

Earthquake Safety

Earthquakes cannot be accurately predicted. Programs in earthquake-prone areas must always be ready for them. The risks from earthquakes include falling objects and destruction of the facility itself. Anything that can move or fall on someone becomes a hazard during an earthquake. According to the Federal Emergency Management Agency (FEMA), most injuries during earthquakes are caused by falling objects, not the movement of the earth during the quake (2006).

Preparation cannot prevent an earthquake, but you can take a variety of measures to minimize destruction and injuries. Secure equipment, gather emergency supplies, locate gas shutoffs, and make plans for sheltering and communicating with families. FEMA has developed *Earthquake Preparedness: What Every Child Care Provider Needs to Know.* This booklet describes the preventive measures that minimize injuries if an earthquake occurs. You can download it from the FEMA website (www.fema.gov/library/viewRecord.do?id=1520).

Part of your program's safety education should be teaching children the drop, cover, and hold on procedure. Follow this procedure at the first sign of the ground shaking. The technique requires you and the children to

1. **drop** to the ground where you are;

2. take **cover**—get under a nearby sturdy table or other piece of furniture; and

3. **hold on** to something sturdy until the shaking stops.

Drop, cover, and hold on is easy for children to learn and should be rehearsed just like other emergency drills.

EARTHQUAKE SAFETY

Goal: We protect children by minimizing risks associated with earthquakes.

❑ Programs check with local experts about the likelihood of earthquakes in the area.

❑ The program conducts earthquake drills monthly.

❑ Teachers practice drop, cover, and hold on with the children at least monthly.

❑ An earthquake kit is prepared and kept at the facility. The kit includes at least a seventy-two-hour supply of food and water, including infant formula, diapers, first aid kit, blankets, whistle, flashlight, portable battery-operated radio and extra batteries, and children's emergency contact information.

❑ All heavy furniture has been secured with brackets or other anchors.

❑ All heavy equipment sits on low shelves or the floor or is secured by straps or anchors.

❑ All overhead light fixtures are securely attached and braced.

❑ All cabinets have latches.

❑ No heavy pictures or mirrors hang above cribs or areas where children sleep.

❑ All wheeled carts or bookcases have locking wheels and are locked in place.

❑ A building contractor has checked the facility and repaired any cracks in the ceiling or foundation. Inflexible utility connections have been replaced with flexible ones. Any loose wiring has been repaired or replaced. Electrical and plumbing connections are in good condition.

❑ If the facility uses natural gas, the building has an automatic, earthquake-activated natural gas shutoff valve. If not, the program has consulted a local building contractor to determine the feasibility of installing such a device. Shutoff valves prevent fires caused by breaks in natural gas pipes after earthquakes. A plan is in place to install a system if possible.

❏ Staff members know how to shut off electricity, gas, and water if necessary.

❏ Teachers practice evacuating and sheltering children in case of an earthquake.

Did you know? If you live in an earthquake-prone area, you can easily become complacent about quakes. Remember that young children have not had as much experience as you and may need reassurance even when very small tremors occur.

❏ Records of the program's earthquake emergency practices are available.

❏ The records are reviewed annually to find opportunities to improve practices.

Medical Emergency Preparedness

Most injuries in programs are minor, but even minor injuries require prompt and effective attention. Teachers need to pay close attention to injured children's physical and emotional needs. Emotional needs, though less visible, can be as much or more important than physical ones. Sometimes when children are hurt, they are actually more scared than physically injured.

First aid training helps you respond to a wide range of medical emergencies, including cuts, scrapes, and choking. Cleaning and bandaging a child's "ouchie" may seem like a commonsense skill, but first aid can be complex. It requires specialized training. The American Red Cross and other organizations offer first aid training specifically designed for early childhood professionals. Many licensing agencies require some or all of the people working with children to have first aid training from a qualified provider.

Cardiopulmonary resuscitation, or **CPR,** is a critically important skill for anyone working with children. Being able to administer CPR can make the difference in saving a child's life in an accident like an electrocution or a drowning. Only adults who have been certified to conduct CPR should do so. All adults working with young children should be certified in pediatric CPR, which is specific to the needs of children. Pediatric CPR training includes techniques for unblocking airways in cases of choking and rescue breathing.

First aid and CPR skills require regular refreshing. Recommendations change from time to time when medical experts learn new or improved ways to treat children. For example, CPR recommendations from the American Heart Association changed in 2010, reinforcing the need for regular retraining.

Note: Items addressed in Standard Precautions (see pages 107–9) also apply to Medical Emergency Preparedness.

MEDICAL EMERGENCY PREPARATION

Goal: We are prepared to protect children's health and safety during medical emergencies.

❑ All adults working in the program have been certified in first aid and pediatric CPR.

Did you know? If you have not recently completed training in first aid and CPR, now is an excellent time to refresh your skills. Without regular education and practice, your skills can become rusty and out of date. The changes to the CPR procedure made by the American Heart Association in 2010 significantly alter the order in which chest compressions, airway clearing, and rescue breathing are administered. The changes adjust the ratio of chest compressions to ventilations to 30:2 (AAP, APHA, and NRC 2011). Most CPR certifications must be renewed every two or three years, depending on the organization that issues the certification, but you can refresh your skills more frequently in classes available in most communities for parents and child care providers.

❑ A standardized form is used to communicate with families about injuries, even minor ones.

❑ Records are on file of all injuries sustained by children while participating in the program.

❑ The records are reviewed annually to find opportunity to improve supervision, replace hazardous equipment, and take other preventive measures.

Section 20

Injury Prevention

As a teacher of young children, you can prevent many injuries to young children directly and indirectly. Most injuries sustained by young children are unintentional. They have accidents that result in bumps and bruises. Sadly, some injuries sustained by young children are both intentional and preventable.

Child abuse injuries include ones arising from **shaken baby syndrome** and other forms of abuse. Abuse affects thousands of children and their families each year. These injuries and deaths are preventable, and you play an important role in ensuring that they do not happen.

Use these three strategies to protect the well-being of young children:

First, you can do a lot to prevent abuse from occurring in your program by implementing the items in the checklist that follows. Many of the recommendations included in the checklist, such as background checks and training, may be required by your licensing agency. Others are best practices you should use to benefit you, the children, and the families you serve.

Second, you can provide support for families to minimize abuse occurring in children's homes. Providing support for families can significantly reduce harm to children.

Third, you can learn to recognize the signs of abuse so children receive immediate treatment when abuse occurs. Because you work with children, you are a mandated reporter. This means you are legally obligated to report any suspicions that a child is being abused inside your program or outside of it, for example, at home.

Sudden unexplained infant deaths are often not the result of child abuse. Sometimes the causes of these deaths cannot be explained. Early childhood professionals are in a unique position to protect children from **Sudden Infant Death Syndrome (SIDS)** and other sudden deaths. First, evaluate and improve practices in the program to promote safe sleep. Second, help protect children's health and welfare by educating families about the risks of some sleep practices, for example, putting children to sleep on their tummies.

This section will address:

- Preventing child abuse: Early childhood programs are in a powerful position to help prevent child abuse.

- Preventing **shaken baby syndrome**: Shaking infants violently can cause head trauma and death. This form of child abuse is entirely preventable.

- Safe sleep: Infants are at risk from Sudden Unexplained Infant Death (SUID), including Sudden Infant Death Syndrome (SIDS).

Preventing Child Abuse

Most children are supported by a community of loving and supportive adults who nurture their development and help them thrive. Sometimes the adults who love and care for children become overwhelmed by stress, isolation, poor parenting skills, bad habits, or their own histories. They make choices that lead to the abuse of children. Early childhood programs are uniquely well suited to prevent **child abuse** and neglect.

Even under the most stringent definitions, more than 1.25 million children are estimated to experience maltreatment each year in the United States. Of these children, most are victims of neglect (61 percent), but a large number are victims of abuse. Most of the abused children suffer physical abuse (58 percent). About 25 percent experience sexual abuse, and 25 percent experience emotional abuse. Children's biological parents are responsible for most abuse. Only sexual abuse is more likely to be perpetrated by adults other than children's biological parents. The severity of abuse increases when the abuser is someone other than a parent (Sedlak et al. 2010).

You can help to prevent child abuse by ensuring that it never occurs in your program. Child abuse is uncommon in child care facilities, but it does happen. Caring for children can be demanding and stressful. But you can put many precautions in place to reduce the risk that you or one of your coworkers will hurt a child while feeling stressed.

As a mandated reporter of child abuse and neglect, you are a valuable source of information about potential child abuse and neglect. You play a vital role in the child protection system. You must report suspicions of child abuse or neglect to the local child protection agency or other responsible party as required by your regulatory agency. You are not required to determine if abuse or neglect has occurred. Become familiar with the regulations and resources in your community so you will know what organizations or agencies are responsible for collecting and acting on reports of child abuse.

You also play an important role in preventing child abuse by serving as a support for families. Part 3 of this book addresses family stress, your role in building resilience among children, and providing family support and education.

PREVENTING CHILD ABUSE

Goal: We protect children from the risks associated with child abuse inside and outside of our program.

❑ Comprehensive background checks, including FBI clearances that require fingerprinting, are obtained for each adult working in the program before the person's first day of work. This includes volunteers and vendors.

Did you know? Not all states require the same level of background check. It is important not to rely on a minimal background check when considering children's safety. Comprehensive background checks include FBI clearance and fingerprints, which better identify criminal histories of anyone who has lived in a different state or under an alias. Checks should also include sex offender registries and child abuse and neglect registries. Alarmingly, many states don't currently require this of child care programs. Comprehensive background checks do take more time and are slightly more expensive, but considering the alternatives, they are certainly worth the commitment. For more information on comprehensive background checks or information on obtaining them, refer to your local Child Care Resource and Referral (CCR&R) or NACCRRA at www.naccrra.org/public-policy/policy-issues/background-checks.

❑ References and employment history are checked for each new hire before the first day of working with children.

❑ A minimum of three references are checked and documented in writing. Professional references are used. References from family members are not accepted.

❑ A written policy is followed that describes the forms of guidance and **discipline** permitted in the program. (Refer to part 3 for specifics about best practices on child guidance.)

❑ The policy is reviewed with all staff members working with young children before they start working with children. A signed copy of the policy is retained in each adult's file.

❑ Teachers are trained in appropriate forms of guidance and interactions with young children before they work with children.

❑ Teachers are trained to identify the signs of child abuse or neglect before working with young children and regularly thereafter. The trainer is the program's child care health consultant or another health professional designated by the regulatory agency.

❑ Teachers are trained to report suspected child abuse and neglect by the program's child care health consultant or another health professional designated by our regulatory agency. The training must be completed before teachers work with young children and regularly thereafter.

❑ Every effort is made to have at least two adults working with groups of children at all times.

❑ Mirrors, windows, and open doors are used to make all children's spaces easily observable.

❑ Rooms are kept at least partially lit by natural or electric light whenever children are present, including naptime rooms.

❑ Teachers working with young children take regular breaks.

❑ Teachers who work alone with young children are offered frequent breaks and opportunities for support during challenging times of the day.

❑ Teachers who feel frustrated, stressed, or angry are encouraged to ask for help or for a break from working with young children.

Did you know? You must be able to recognize signs of stress in your own behavior and that of your coworkers. Think about how you typically feel when you become angry, frustrated, or out of control. You may feel tightness in your chest or notice that your hands become tight fists. You may feel warm, or your face may flush. Whatever the signs, these are cues that you need a moment to regroup and regain control of your emotions and reactions. Being honest about your feelings and taking action to prevent an out-of-control behavior helps to ensure that children in your program do not become victims of a tragic action.

❑ The program provides parent-education resources for families.

❑ The program is familiar with community resources that can support families experiencing stress or other risk factors for abuse or neglect.

Did you know? Many child care programs and teachers don't realize that they play an important role in minimizing child maltreatment or parental stress. The Center for the Study of Social Policy has developed *Strengthening Families: A Guidebook for Early Childhood Programs*, an excellent resource that describes your role in preventing child abuse through working with children and families. The report and other helpful resources are available online (http://www.cssp.org/reform/strengthening-families).

Preventing Shaken Baby Syndrome

When you hold infants, you are typically careful to support their heads. This is because infants are still developing neck and other muscles that help them hold their heads in place. Infants count on you to be gentle and supportive. They are extremely susceptible to head trauma.

One form of child abuse that affects approximately 1,000 infants each year is **shaken baby syndrome**. The number of cases is difficult to determine, but estimates range from 600 to 1,400 cases each year. Approximately 20 percent of shaken baby syndrome cases are fatal. Nonfatal cases experience a range of impact from mild, such as learning disabilities and behavior changes, to severe, such as profound mental and developmental retardation, paralysis, blindness, and permanent vegetative state (National Center on Shaken Baby Syndrome 2011).

Shaken baby syndrome is entirely preventable. Most events leading to shaken baby syndrome are the result of adults' inappropriate overreactions to infants' inconsolable crying or from patterns of abuse in the adults' own families (CDC 2012).

You can play an important part in preventing shaken baby syndrome. First, ensure that the shaking of infants never occurs in your program. For example, you can ensure that teachers who appear frustrated are given regular breaks, or you can offer or participate in training for infant teachers to help them understand infants' needs. You can also help families to understand the risks of shaken baby syndrome and the resources available to support them in managing stress appropriately. Second, you can be aware of signs indicating that a child has been the victim of shaking. While this awareness may not prevent the abuse, it can help ensure that infants receive immediate and potentially lifesaving treatment.

PREVENTING SHAKEN BABY SYNDROME

Goal: We protect children from the risks of shaken baby syndrome.

❑ Teachers are trained to recognize the symptoms of shaken baby syndrome and to prevent it. They are trained by the program's child care health consultant or another health professional as required by the regulatory agency.

❑ Teachers are trained in several methods for consoling infants and meeting their individual needs. The trainings are conducted by the program's child care health consultant or another expert in infant care.

❑ We have a policy that requires teachers to report suspected instances of shaken baby syndrome in the same way they report other child abuse suspicions.

❑ Teachers who work with infants are routinely observed by other adults and the program's child care health consultant.

❑ Teachers who work with infants take regular breaks.

❑ Teachers who are feeling stressed are encouraged to ask for help or ask for a break from working with infants.

❑ Our program provides educational materials to families to help them avoid shaking their infants at home.

❑ Our staff members are familiar with resources in the community for families experiencing stress. We share parenting information with families.

Did you know? If you are not familiar with parent education resources in your community, investigate. Start with your local school district. The early childhood special education program often has information about parenting education for parents of typically developing children and those with special needs. Your child care health consultant can also help you identify resources for parent support and education. Part 3 of this book also contains additional recommendations you can use to help families manage stress.

Safe Sleep

Few sights are more peaceful than sleeping babies. Sleep is as necessary to development as nutrition and exercise. During sleep, infants rest their muscles and prepare for the active exploration that takes place when they're awake. Most of the time, they get ten or more hours of sleep each day without incident. Sometimes tragedy occurs, and infants do not wake from sleep.

Approximately 4,600 infants die suddenly each year. These infants are not ill, and in some cases the immediate cause of death is unexplained. Many of the **Sudden Unexplained Infant Deaths (SUIDs)** are later attributed to suffocation, poisoning, hypothermia, hyperthermia, or abuse. These deaths are preventable (Shapiro-Mendoza 2012).

About half of the SUIDs are attributed to **Sudden Infant Death Syndrome (SIDS)**. Even after thorough investigation, these cannot be explained. SIDS has no known cause, but certain preventive measures have been effective in reducing its incidence. SIDS is most likely to occur when an infant is between two and four months of age. Ninety percent of cases occur before six months of age (Shapiro-Mendoza 2012).

Since the discovery of a link between sleep position and SIDS, parents and teachers have been urged to place infants on their backs to sleep. This change in practice has resulted in a dramatic drop in the incidence of SIDS deaths (Task Force on Sudden Infant Death Syndrome 2011). The National Institute of Child Health and Human Development's long-running Back to Sleep campaign has educated parents and teachers on the importance of putting infants on their backs for sleeping. Nevertheless, SIDS remains a serious threat to infants. Over two thousand deaths in the United States each year are attributed to SIDS. A small percentage of these occur in child care programs (Shapiro-Mendoza 2012).

Many of the same precautions that seem to reduce the risk of infant death from SIDS also help to prevent deaths from other causes, like suffocation. Safe sleep and back to sleep campaigns often address a variety of precautions to ensure the safety of infants.

SAFE SLEEP

Goal: We protect children from the risks associated with SIDS and other sudden infant deaths.

❑ Teachers are trained on how to prevent SIDS before working with infants and every two years thereafter. The training is given by the program's child care health consultant or other health professional as required by the regulatory agency.

❑ Teachers place infants to sleep on their backs unless written directions from the infant's physician specify another position.

❑ Infants are placed on their backs even if they can roll over on their own.

❑ Placards indicating that infants are able to roll over or have physician permission to sleep on their tummies are posted on cribs to eliminate potential teacher mistakes.

❑ Infants are placed in the crib with their feet near the foot of the crib.

❑ Blankets are not used unless requested by parents.

❑ Blankets, when used in response to parent direction, are tucked into the sides of the crib, between the crib mattress and crib sides. They are pulled up to the infant's chest, and the infant's arms are placed on top of the blanket. Adults in the program never cover infants' faces with blankets, pillows, hats, or other items.

Did you know? It can be difficult for parents to think of their infant sleeping in a crib without a blanket, even if it is a safe sleep practice. Some programs have begun recommending sleep sacks as an alternative to blankets. Sleep sacks are wearable blankets that won't cover a baby's face while he sleeps.

❑ Teachers are careful to be sure that infant clothes are not tight at the neck. Bibs are removed when infants are not eating.

❑ We support the use of pacifiers.

Did you know? Medical experts are unsure why the incidence of SIDS is lower among infants who use pacifiers. Because this is the case, you should offer a pacifier to infants as they move into sleep. If an infant does not use the pacifier or the pacifier falls out of the infant's mouth during sleep, simply remove it from the crib. Never force an infant to use a pacifier.

❑ Infant cribs do not have bumper pads.

❑ Infant cribs do not have pillows, soft toys, or blankets that are not in use.

❑ Infant cribs do not have mobiles or other toys with strings within infants' reach.

❑ There are no window blind cords or other dangling strings within three feet of infant cribs.

❑ Infants are placed in cribs without bottles, sippy cups, loose blankets, pillows, or soft toys.

❑ Our program shares information with families about preventing SIDS and other sudden infant deaths.

Did you know? The American Academy of Pediatrics, American Public Health Association, and National Resource Center for Health and Safety in Child Care and Early Education have gathered all of their recommendations for safe sleep practices and the reduction of risk from SIDS and suffocation on one document. You can access this helpful document online at http://nrckids.org/SPINOFF/SAFESLEEP/SafeSleep.pdf.

Section 21

Security

Children must feel safe and secure to thrive. For the most part, you create a feeling of security for the children in your care by being available and responsive to their needs. Your presence, your reassuring tone, your responsiveness, and your involvement in their daily activities reassure them. They know they can safely explore their environment, try new things, and learn about the world around them using their emerging skills. Without a sense of security, children do not develop confidence or the ability to take appropriate risks or solve problems.

Besides emotional security, you provide physical security for the children in your care. You create and maintain an environment that minimizes risks and threats. In some cases, you keep children secure from their own lack of judgment and experience. For example, you may place a bell or buzzer on an outside door so you know if a child leaves the building when you are not looking. By doing this, you protect that child from traffic or other hazards found outside.

Some of the security measures you develop are designed to address the complex nature of today's families. For example, children in your care may have more than one residence and may divide their time between parents who are no longer living together. Child custody arrangements require your attention to detail and clear communication to avoid confusion for you, the family members, and, most important, the child.

This section will address:

- Building security: Whether the program takes place in a home or a commercial building, there are many things you can do to enhance the security of the facility. Some security measures are structural, such as the use of fences. Other security measures are practices that you will follow, such as checking the identification of people who pick up children.

Building Security

Child care facilities come in a wide variety of shapes, sizes, and configurations. Some programs are held in a family's residential home; others are located in commercial buildings designed for the care of young children. Each of the many types of facilities has merits and challenges, and security of the facility must be attended to in all of them.

Child care facilities have special security challenges that other buildings or homes may not. Many adults, including family members, vendors, and regulatory persons, come and go frequently. Programs want to be welcoming but must balance openness with reasonable precautions for the children's security.

The children who attend your program may not always appreciate the need for them to remain safely within the facility's grounds. Without precautions in place, children may leave the building without adequate supervision. Young children have been known to wander outside of the play yard through an open gate without regard for nearby traffic or other hazards.

Commercial facilities may have security systems to support providers in providing a safe environment. Even when such a system is available, nothing replaces the vigilance of the adults working in the program.

BUILDING SECURITY

Goal: The design and maintenance of our facility help keep children safe. Our practices protect children's security.

❑ Automatic sensors on all outside doors trigger chimes or buzzers to alert staff members when a door is opened.

❑ A fence surrounds the entire outdoor play area. It has no gaps through which children can leave the area.

❑ If a gate is part of the fence, the latch is out of children's reach.

❑ Families are required to indicate in writing who can pick up their child.

❑ Families may not authorize minors to pick up children.

❑ We enforce a policy requiring picture identification for anyone picking up children, other than custodial parents or guardians.

❑ Families are not allowed to authorize new pickup persons over the telephone, by e-mail, or by other electronic communication, such as text messages.

❑ If a parent authorizes a person to pick up their child repeatedly, but they are not on the official authorized list, the parent is asked to add the person to the list.

❑ Our program asks for information about child custody when families enroll. Court documents affecting custody must be submitted then, including current restraining orders, divorce decrees with custody instructions, and/or adoption judgments.

❑ A copy of any child custody order that prohibits one family member from having access to a child enrolled in the program must be on file. Verbal directions are not followed. Proof of custody is required when the family enrolls.

❑ Staff members receive training on the program's pickup procedures during their **orientation** before working with children and regularly thereafter.

❑ Our schedule is planned so that adults working in the program become familiar with family members who pick up and drop off children.

❑ Staff members follow a consent for safe departure policy by calling another person on the authorized list if the person picking up the child appears unsafe to release the child to.

Did you know? A consent for safe departure policy is an important policy to have and to practice. This policy addresses the response you should have when you don't feel it is safe releasing a child to the parent or authorized guardian. You may feel unsafe for a variety of reasons: perhaps you heard the adult threatening abuse or you suspect the adult has been drinking. It can be difficult to tell a parent or authorized guardian that you cannot release a child to her because you don't feel it's safe to do so. Role-playing this scenario can ease teachers' anxiety. This situation doesn't occur often, but when it does, children count on teachers to do what is necessary to protect them.

❑ Our program provides families with a written policy (safe departure policy) on procedures to be followed if no one (including persons on authorized lists) picks up the child.

❑ The front door area is never left unattended during arrival and departure times.

❑ Families are trained not to hold the door open for unknown persons attempting to enter the facility.

❑ Substitutes, volunteers, or temporary staff members are not allowed to work alone with children.

Did you know? Departure time can be a very busy part of the day. This is also when you are likely to be most fatigued from a full day of activity with the children. Careful planning for end-of-the-day activities can help you navigate this part of the day successfully. Plan a few activities the children can do with minimal supervision from you. Avoid activities like water play that you must attend to closely. This way, you can be somewhat free to interact with families as they arrive and reunite with children. Your presence and attention can help smooth these interactions and help to end the day on a positive note.

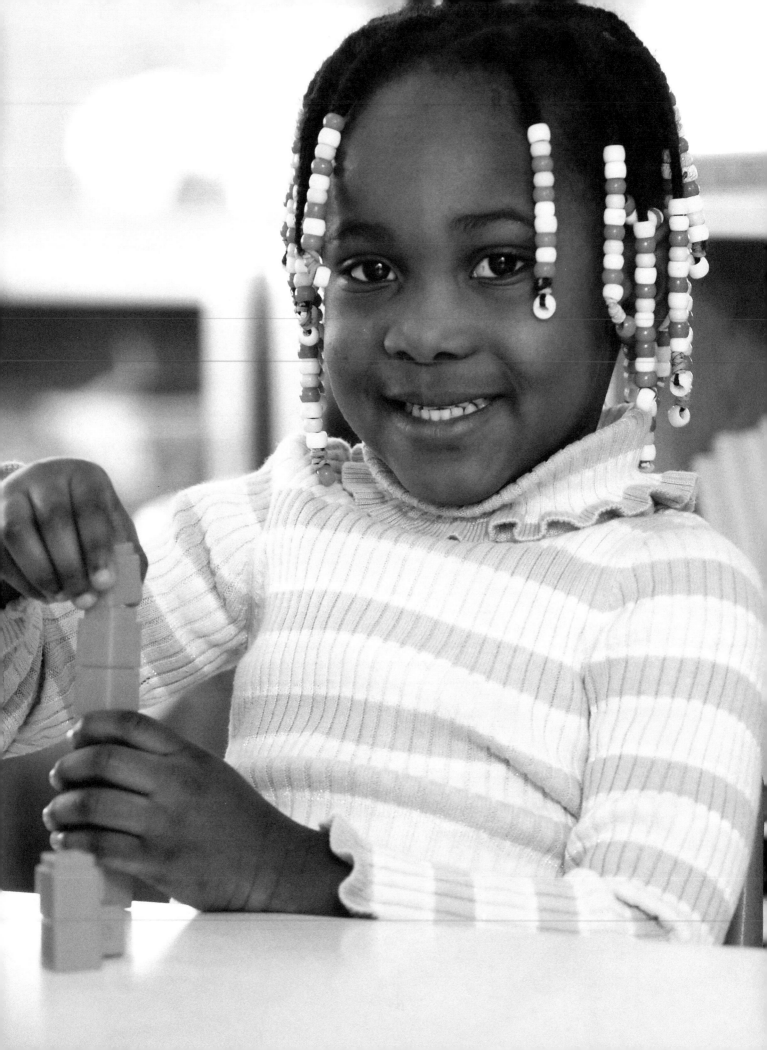

Part 6

Leadership

Early childhood programs are led by individuals who are responsible for hiring and supervising staff members, financial management, marketing and enrollment, communicating with families, development of policies, procedures, and training, and much, much more. These leaders are called *directors, executive directors, site coordinators,* or other titles. Sometimes these leaders are also the **primary caregiver** or teacher.

The governance of the program may involve many people, a few people, or one person who owns and operates the program. In a family child care program, the program leader may also be the program owner and the teacher working directly with children each day. In other child care and early childhood programs, the program leader may report to a board of directors, a parent council, a principal, or another level of authority in a larger organization.

The heart of every early childhood program is serving children and their families. Most early childhood programs describe their work and their goals in a written mission statement. Program leaders use the mission statement as a guide for making good decisions. Your mission may include a statement about your interest in promoting children's health and wellness. This aspect of your mission may drive many of your leadership decisions.

Program leaders are essential in promoting and maintaining quality practices in early care and education. Research indicates that program leadership is linked to quality of care and to positive child outcomes. Gwen Morgan (2000) explains:

> Anyone who has ever worked in, or enrolled a child in, a good early childhood program knows that leadership is critical. Administrative actions create a healthy organization that functions as a supportive community for children and staff. The director, often working within the framework set by a sponsoring organization, makes the decisions that create the conditions for good child outcomes. (160)

The work of leading the program has a significant impact on the overall health and wellness of children. For example, program leaders may not serve lunch, but they may be the ones creating the budget for food purchases or developing the policies about what types of foods will be served in the program. Leadership influences children and families through the policies developed, the way information is gathered and shared, and the planning and budgeting of programs.

You may think that leadership is merely administrative, characterized by developing, communicating, and enforcing policies that govern the program. In reality, leadership is much more dynamic than this. Program leaders perform a wide variety of tasks that directly and indirectly impact the care that children receive. For example, leaders perform personnel management tasks such as hiring and training. They also perform financial management tasks such as purchasing supplies and overseeing budgets. All of these tasks can be organized into categories of work that provide a picture of the breadth of the leadership role. Morgan (2000, 41) describes eight areas in which program leaders must demonstrate competency to provide high-quality programs:

1. The ability to plan and implement a developmentally appropriate care and education program for children and families.

2. The ability to develop and maintain an effective organization.

3. The ability to plan and implement administrative systems that effectively carry out the program's mission, goals, and objectives.

4. The ability to administer effectively a program of personnel management and staff member development.

5. The ability to foster good community relations and to influence the child care policy that affects the program.

6. The ability to maintain and develop the physical facility.

7. The legal knowledge necessary for effective management.

8. The ability to apply financial management tools.

From this list, you can see that being a program leader is a big, complex job. It has great influence on children, families, and other adults working in the program. Program leaders can take great pride in knowing that their efforts can positively affect many people for long periods of time.

Effective program leaders continuously work to fulfill the mission of the program; they evaluate and reevaluate policies and practices and partner with families and staff members to negotiate dilemmas that face all programs. In practice, the leadership role often includes shared decision making and collaboration. These practices allow leaders to negotiate differences of priorities and to create programs in which children and families thrive.

In the sections that follow, the focus is on aspects of leadership that affect the health and safety of programs. These include process features, like selecting and evaluating staff members, and structural features, like maintaining facilities. The focus is on health and safety aspects of leadership, not the full range of activities associated with leading an early childhood program. Nonetheless, a wide range of topics are addressed, because health and safety are intertwined in many aspects of programs. Addressing some of these health and safety considerations can have a positive impact on other areas outside the scope of this book. For example, one checklist addresses employee **orientation** and recommends a robust program of orientation. Such orientations affect children's health and safety. They can also contribute to communication with families, their satisfaction, and the learning programs offered to the children.

Section 22

Communicating with Families about Health, Safety, and Fitness

Amy Baker and Lynn Manfredi/Petitt state, "When adults have trusting relationships with plenty of give-and-take and care is seamless, children reap the benefits" (2004, 10). Although positive relationships are important, they do not always develop easily or quickly. To help develop and maintain positive relationships, program leaders develop materials, policies, procedures, and communications systems. They also model effective **interpersonal** dynamics.

To help families select care that meets their needs and matches their philosophy of child rearing, you must clearly describe your program's mission, philosophy, policies, and practices. These important statements also help to minimize potential confusion or misunderstandings while you and the families work together.

You can communicate written policies and procedures to families in a variety of ways. Most programs create a handbook or booklet to share with families when they enroll. Written materials are very helpful in creating clear expectations. Written policies should also be reviewed regularly and updated as needed.

A comprehensive family handbook helps you begin communicating with families, but it's only one tool. Besides written statements that define and describe the program, you are responsible for maintaining regular communication with families. In early childhood programs, family members visit frequently. Most parents drop off their children and pick them up at the end of the day. This pattern creates many chances for informal conversations and develops relationships, builds trust, and supports problem solving.

Informal communications like daily conversations are important for sharing information about children and your program. More formal or planned opportunities to share information with families include daily notes, newsletters, parent meetings, and conferences. All of these provide ways to get to know families, share information about children's development, and alert families to changes in policies or procedures. One form of formal communication is the intake meeting, which occurs before children begin in the program. It's a wonderful chance to get to know more about children and their families. It is also a chance to begin developing the very important relationship you will have with them.

This section will address:

- Written policies and statements of practice: Well-organized and effective early childhood programs need policies on many health and wellness topics.

- Routine communications with families: Communication helps to build relationships that are essential to high-quality care for children.

- Intake meetings: Holding a face-to-face meeting with the family before a child's first day in the program starts the relationship and provides time to share information and answer questions.

- Community resources: Connecting families to community resources gives them information that can greatly enhance health and well-being. It also demonstrates to families your interest in them and your expertise as an early childhood professional.

- Decision making: Myriad decisions must be made when caring for children. While families are the primary decision makers for their children, you will share in that responsibility.

Written Policies and Statements of Practice

In early childhood programs, **policies** serve as written standards for the well-being and safety of families and staff members. Programs use policies to guide their decision making and actions. Most programs have written policies that can be communicated easily and that minimize confusion.

Program policies can be developed in a number of ways. Some policies may be required by child care licensing rules or regulatory agencies. Others may result from your program's mission. For example, a program with a mission that specifies the inclusion of children with special needs will have many policies about enrolling children with special needs and how their needs will be addressed. Still other policies are designed to promote the smooth operation of the program. For example, your program may have policies that address when fees must be paid or how information about **immunizations** is collected.

Policies often specify that you use particular practices. Practices are the actions carried out in programs. For example, you may have a policy to enroll children only after obtaining certain information from the family. Based on this policy, you can adopt the practice of holding an intake meeting with each family before the child attends the program.

Well-developed policies stand the test of time and change infrequently. You want to provide opportunities for those affected by a policy to learn about the policy and share their concerns about it before it is enacted or changed. Providing this due-process opportunity strengthens and encourages support of the policy.

Programs often communicate policies and practices in written form in a family handbook or manual. Increasingly, policy statements are found on a program's website or in other electronic documents.

WRITTEN POLICIES

Goal: We develop written health and wellness policies and communicate them to the families we serve.

❏ The program provides a family handbook or similar document that describes the policies affecting the health and wellness of children and families.

❏ A copy of the handbook describing our policies is given to all families when they enroll.

❏ A copy of the handbook and all policies are given to teachers.

❏ Families are required to state in writing that they have received, read, and understood the program's policies.

❏ Written policy documents are given to families in their primary language.

❏ Our handbook has been reviewed and approved by the program's child care health consultant and a legal adviser.

❏ Our handbook is reviewed annually by the program's leadership and the child care health consultant.

❏ Our policies and handbook can be quickly changed when recommendations from health organizations, licensing agencies, or others require changes in practices.

❏ Our handbook contains a written complaint procedure that explains how issues can be solved jointly between families and the program.

❏ New written copies of the policies are provided to all families when changes in policies are made.

❏ When advisable, family meetings are held to discuss new policies before they are enacted.

Did you know? Think about the language you are choosing to express new policy. Whenever possible, choose positive language that reinforces what is permitted and encouraged. Focus on the goal or the why of the policy. For example, a policy about bringing toys from home can be stated in a positive way: *We provide all of the toys and materials your child will need during the day in our program. We ask that you leave your child's own toys at home so he or she can enjoy them there without concern about sharing with other children or any damages to the toys.*

GUIDANCE POLICIES AND PROCEDURES

Goal: We protect children's health and wellness by developing and communicating policies and procedures about child guidance.

❑ The family handbook describes the program's policies and procedures related to child guidance.

Did you know? Child guidance, or **discipline**, is an emotional subject for many families. Families may struggle with the best approach to guide their child's behavior. Often they have only their own childhood experiences to rely on. Child guidance is a great topic for parent information and education. Just remember, if you offer a parent session on this topic, be prepared for a big turnout!

❑ Our policies restrict the use of time-outs or practice of isolating children as a form of discipline.

❑ Our policies and procedures clearly prohibit corporal **punishment** by staff members, volunteers, or family members on the premises and during any program-sponsored events, including off-site activities.

❑ Our policies and procedures clearly explain the guidance or discipline methods used in the program to support children's development of social and emotional skills and to reduce challenging behaviors. (Refer to part 3 for more information on child guidance.)

❑ The procedures clearly explain
    ❑ how staff members respond to repeated or severe challenging behaviors
    ❑ how families will be given reports about these behaviors
    ❑ the expectation that families will be involved in addressing the behaviors

❑ The policies explain the specific conditions that can cause a child to be excluded from the program (for example, severe or repeated challenging behaviors).

TRANSITION POLICIES AND PROCEDURES

Goal: We protect children's health and wellness by developing and communicating policies on transitions in our program.

❑ Our family handbook contains policies that address transitions between groups in the program.

❑ Our policies specify that children move from one care group to another (for example, from an infant to a toddler care group) based on developmental readiness rather than a birth date or a single skill, such as potty training.

❑ Our policies specify that staff members plan transitions in advance and in collaboration with families.

❑ Our policies explain that staff members encourage families to discuss the transition with their child. Information is available to help them talk about the transition with their child.

❑ Our policies describe the practice of asking children and families to visit the new environment and establish a relationship with the new teacher before a transition begins.

❑ Our policies state that when staff members plan transitions to a new care group within the same facility, they take place gradually over at least several weeks.

❑ Our policies explain that children's transitions are made easier by allowing comfort items, such as blankets or a favorite book, to move with the child.

❑ Our policies include information on how staff members work with local schools and families. Together, we plan children's transitions to kindergarten or another child care facility.

Did you know? Transitions from one group to another can be challenging for children and their families. Transitions occur oftentimes because that's simply how they've always been done. But are they necessary? Consider minimizing the number of transitions experienced by children and eliminate unnecessary changes. Section 9 in part 3 of this book has additional information about transitions and their impact on children.

FOOD AND NUTRITION POLICIES

Goal: We protect children's health and wellness by developing and communicating policies on food and nutrition in the program.

❏ Our handbook contains policies and procedures addressing food and children's nutrition. This information is reviewed with the family at the time of enrollment.

❏ Our policies require families to provide information from their medical care provider describing any physical limitations or conditions affecting their child's nutrition requirements or foods (for example, food allergies).

❏ Our handbook explains the procedures that will be used if allergic reactions occur.

❏ Our handbook invites families to provide information about personal, cultural, or religious preferences affecting their child's foods or eating (for example, the family is vegetarian).

❏ Our handbook includes information about the program's policy of providing information about nutrition during pregnancy to pregnant families.

❏ Our handbook includes information about the program's policy and procedures to actively support breast-feeding. It explains the program's provisions for families who choose to continue breast-feeding while their child is enrolled in the program.

❏ Our handbook explains the healthy procedures teachers use when feeding infants.

❏ Our handbook explains the procedures for **family-style dining** as well as other practices that encourage healthy eating habits.

❏ Our policies require meals or snacks provided by families for children to be healthy and balanced.

❏ Our policies require that foods provided by families for special events or celebrations be **nutritious** and meet healthy food guidelines. They must be commercially prepared if they are to be shared among the children. For example, if food is brought to the program for a birthday celebration, it must be commercially prepared.

❏ Our policies do not allow foods from fast-food restaurants to be brought to the program for children's meals, snacks, or special events.

❏ Our program provides information about children's allergies that affect what food can be brought to the program. We have a designated way to update this information routinely.

❑ Our program has nutritious food on hand to supplement children's meals brought from home if needed. Food brought from home or supplied by other sources is stored safely, including refrigeration when needed.

❑ Our policies require that anyone handling food has been trained in safe procedures.

Bonus Checklist

❑ Our program's child care health consultant has reviewed and approved our food and nutrition policies and procedures.

> **Did you know?** Review part 1 of this book for in-depth information about nutrition and food in early childhood programs.

PHYSICAL PLAY AND ACTIVITY POLICIES

Goal: We protect children's health and wellness by developing and communicating policies on play and physical activity. We describe how play is encouraged by the program.

❑ Our family handbook contains policies that address children's physical play or the program's commitment to encouraging active lifestyles.

❑ The policies exclude these toys and other materials brought from home:
  ❑ war play toys
  ❑ toys or other materials that are age inappropriate
  ❑ toys or devices that emphasize screen time
  ❑ toys, equipment, or materials that have been recalled by the Consumer Products Safety Commission

> **Did you know?** If you do not have policies that address toys from home, consider organizing a small group of parents to work with you to develop the policy. You can describe the program's concerns about toys from home. Then work closely with parents to develop a policy that works for you, the children, and the families you serve. Involving parents in making policies that cross over between the program and home can greatly improve the end results.

❑ Our policies require the program to engage in daily outdoor play and require families to supply outdoor clothing appropriate for active play and the day's weather.

❑ Our handbook states the conditions that may limit outdoor play (for example, air quality or extreme temperatures) and how changes are made to the outdoor play schedule. We share this information with families when changes are made.

❑ Our handbook requires families to provide information from their medical care provider about children's physical limitations and any other conditions that affect active play.

❑ Our handbook invites families to provide information on personal, cultural, or religious practices that affect children's active play.

❑ Our handbook describes any nonprescription medications used in our program to protect children during outdoor play (for example, sunscreens or insect repellants), including a description of products that are acceptable for use. We specify who will provide the products and how and when they will be applied.

❑ Our policies require the use of broad-spectrum sunscreens, or at least SPF 15, used according to the manufacturer's instructions and applied at least fifteen minutes before outdoor play.

❑ Our handbook describes the use of **pesticides** or fertilizers, including our methods for notifying families when they will be used on the premises.

CHILDREN'S HEALTH POLICIES

Goal: We protect children's health and wellness by developing and communicating policies that describe how children's health is addressed by the program.

❑ Our family handbook includes information describing policies and procedures aimed at protecting children's health.

❑ Our policies require parents and other adults to wash their hands before spending time with children during the program day. Parents and other adults must remove their shoes before entering areas where children play on the floors.

❑ Our policies do not permit smoking in the facility, on the grounds, or in vehicles used to transport children during the program day. They also address ways to minimize exposure to **secondhand** and **thirdhand smoke**.

❑ Our policies and procedures require infants to be placed on their backs when sleeping, unless a written direction from the child's physician advises another practice.

❑ Our policies require children's health forms, including a statement of health from children's physicians, to be completed before enrollment. They should be regularly updated.

❑ Our policies require children to be immunized according to the American Academy of Pediatrics' recommended childhood immunization schedule unless exceptions are documented in writing.

❑ Our policies require children to be well in order to attend the program. Specific guidelines explain when children cannot attend the program because of illness.

❑ Our policies explain that staff members can administer routine first aid during accidents or illness. Emergency medical practitioners are used for nonroutine procedures.

❑ Our policies explain that staff members must be able to contact families in emergencies and that contact information must be up-to-date at all times.

❑ Our policies explain that staff members work collaboratively with a child care health consultant to protect children's health and wellness. Families must grant written permission for staff members to share information about their child with the consultant.

❑ Specific policies and practices are in place to guide giving prescription and nonprescription medications. Families are informed about where to leave medications and how medication needs must be documented.

❑ Our policies do not allow families to idle vehicles near doors or windows that open into spaces used by children.

Did you know? Post a sign in your parking area to remind families that cars may not idle near windows that open to the child care space. Parents easily forget this when they are hurried at the beginning and end of the day.

❑ Our policies explain that teachers are mandated reporters of child abuse and neglect.

❑ Our handbook tells families that the program can connect them to community resources on parenting and family stressors.

SECURITY POLICIES AND PROCEDURES

Goal: We protect children's safety, health, and wellness by developing and communicating policies on maintaining security in the program.

❑ Our family handbook includes policies or practices aimed at protecting children's security.

❑ Our policies require families to sign in and out each day when children are dropped off and picked up.

❑ Our policies require families to escort children into the child care space and make contact with the adult in charge before leaving their children.

❑ Our policies require families to notify the program when their children will not attend as scheduled.

❑ Our handbook explains the importance of closing doors and gates when families enter and exit the facility each day.

❑ Our policies require families to specify in writing who may pick up their child from the facility. They must include an emergency contact who can be called when parents cannot be reached. Authorizations communicated by e-mail and over the phone are not acceptable.

❑ Our handbook explains that photo identification is required from anyone who is not immediately known to the adults in charge when picking up a child. The program has a copy of each person's photo identification on file.

Did you know? Most of the time, children are released to the same two or three family members. Other authorized people pick up children only infrequently. Because their presence is rare, you must require their identification before releasing children. It is easy for infrequent visitors to forget about this procedure. Help them by requiring a copy of the photo identification for everyone authorized to pick up a child. Keeping a copy of the photo identification on file ensures that you always have the information you need to check the identity of people picking up children.

❑ Our handbook explains the program's procedure for notifying families and obtaining written permission before any activity or trip requiring transportation of the child. The same is true if the child leaves the program's premises by other means.

❑ Our policies require written documentation of custody orders that may affect who can visit or pick up a child from the program.

❑ Our handbook emphasizes that families must notify the program of any family situation that can affect the child's safety in the program.

❑ The handbook explains the procedures we follow in emergencies, including those that may require **evacuation** from or sheltering within the facility. These may also prevent parents from picking up their child.

❑ The procedures for notifying families when the facility is closed or evacuated and the location of shelters away from the facility are described in our handbook.

Routine Communications with Families

Children benefit directly and indirectly when the adults in their lives have close, caring relationships. When you and the children's families are close, the care you provide to children improves. Great relationships are built on frequent communication.

As a teacher, you benefit from frequent interactions with families. In most programs, family members arrive with the children each morning and pick up their children at the end of the day. When a child attends full-time, you have ten opportunities each week to communicate with a family member! Many teachers in elementary or secondary schools would envy the chance to see the family members of their students so often.

All of these opportunities are meaningful only if you take full advantage of them. Informal time to talk and share information about the child's day builds trust and rapport with family members.

Besides informal conversation each day when children arrive and depart, you have many opportunities for more formal communication. Formal communication tools are used by many programs to strengthen exchanges of information between families and the program. Formal communication is not necessarily more elaborate or more academic than informal communications. It's referred to as *formal* because it's often planned in advance and may have specific goals or requirements. Formal communications include newsletters, parent meetings, and child conferences. These formal communication tools present excellent opportunities to share information about children's health, safety, and **fitness**.

ROUTINE COMMUNICATION WITH FAMILIES

Goal: We share information about children's health, safety, and fitness in a variety of formal and informal ways.

❑ Developing a partnership with parents is a primary goal.

❑ Staff members' schedules and activities are planned to allow time for staff members and adult family members to hold brief conversations during arrival and pickup times.

> **Did you know?** In most programs, you are responsible for supervising children while you are having informal conversations with family members at the beginning and end of each day. If you have a coworker alongside you, consider dividing tasks so one of you can focus on connecting with each family member and the other can keep the child-oriented activities running smoothly. If you are alone with the children, use your activity planning to make yourself as available as possible to family members. Plan activities at the beginning and end of the day that do not require your undivided attention. Position yourself where you can see family members entering the space so you can greet them, even if you are busy with the children.

❑ Written communication (daily note or other tool) is used to exchange information every day about each child's eating, toileting, activities, disposition, and overall wellness. As often as possible, this information is provided in the family's primary language.

❑ Information displays, newsletters, and other communication tools are used regularly (at least once per month) to provide family members with information on children's health and wellness.

❑ Conferences with family members occur at least twice a year. They focus on children's overall development, including their physical health and development and their emotional and social development.

> **Did you know?** If you have never conducted conferences with family members, consider practicing with a friend or coworker. Take the time to role-play a few conversations. Doing so will help ease your nerves and give you confidence. When rehearsing, remember to treat specific information about children as confidential. Use fictitious information during your rehearsal sessions.

❑ Written communication is provided in the primary language used by adult family members.

❏ Interpreters are used for family conferences when family members and teachers do not share a primary language.

❏ Written communication is used to inform family members when children show symptoms of illness or have been injured during the program.

❏ Family members are actively encouraged to share ideas with staff members, especially their child's teacher or **primary caregiver.**

Intake Meetings

At the time a child is enrolled in your program, a great deal of information must be exchanged by you and the child's family. You need to learn enough about the child to provide safe and healthy care, and the adults in the family need to learn how your program works to benefit the children in care.

An intake meeting or conference is one method of exchanging information when a child enrolls or moves to a different classroom or level. This meeting is usually conducted face-to-face and includes adults in the family, the program teacher, and the director of a center-based program. Other support personnel or practitioners may also be included, especially if the enrolling child has special needs.

Intake meetings are a chance to get to know one another and to learn about preferences and expectations. They also are a time to discuss the program's policies and practices. Even if the family toured the program before enrolling, a great deal remains to be discussed to ensure a smooth transition into the program. The intake meeting is a great way to begin developing a relationship with the whole family. The most effective intake meetings provide plenty of time for family members to talk about their needs, interests, and concerns.

INTAKE MEETING

Goal: We ensure children's safe and healthy care by conducting intake meetings when each new family enrolls and when children transition between care groups.

❏ Our policies require an intake meeting before a child's first day in the program or a new classroom.

❏ Adult family members and at least the child's teacher are included in the intake meeting.

❏ Family members are informed that the goal of the intake meeting is to begin to develop a relationship that will support their child's development.

❏ If necessary, an interpreter is present so family members can receive information in their primary language.

❏ Family members receive written information (for example, a family handbook) in advance of the meeting so they are prepared for discussion and questions. They must acknowledge in writing that they have received the information.

❏ Program policies that emphasize children's health and wellness are discussed at the intake meetings. These include the following:
  ❏ Families' priorities and preferences are discussed.
  ❏ The program's open-door policy is explained.
  ❏ Opportunities for involvement are shared.
  ❏ Nutritional plans for infants are completed if relevant.

❏ Family members are encouraged to ask questions. Time is allowed for questions about the program and its philosophy, policies, and practices.

❏ Staff members conducting intake meetings have been trained to do so. They know how to welcome families and help them feel at ease.

Did you know? When conducting intake meetings, remember that family members may feel nervous. They may still be unsure about their decision to enroll their child in an early childhood program. Your role is to support them as well as their child. Most parents appreciate your **active listening** and **empathy**. These go a long way toward easing any tensions families may have.

❏ Newly enrolled families are introduced to other families in the program.

❏ Newly enrolled families are connected with a mentor family.

Community Resources

Children's health, safety, and fitness needs can sometimes be complex. They may require resources well beyond those available within your program. Very few early childhood programs have services that meet all of the needs families may have. Collecting information about local resources for families can help you connect families to services that your program does not offer.

Families may not be aware of the many resources in their community. Because you work with many families and possess expert knowledge, families expect you to serve as a link to resources that can benefit them. You must become aware of resources in the community that can support families and help to meet children's needs. While this may seem like an added burden to your already busy schedule, in the end it will support your efforts to provide children and their families with opportunities that help them thrive.

The types of resources from which families can benefit vary broadly. Some families may need or want family education or parenting resources. Others may be interested in resources that help them to maintain their health and wellness, such as child care assistance, food programs, or medical care programs.

Your knowledge of local resources can also help families make decisions that greatly benefit their children. For example, helping a family to connect with a local immunization clinic also protects a child from serious illness. Helping a family connect to a **medical home** may improve their child's medical care throughout childhood and encourage healthy habits for the child's lifetime.

COMMUNITY RESOURCES

Goal: We connect families to resources in the community that support children's health and wellness.

- ❏ Our program helps families without regular health care providers find resources that meet their children's health needs.

- ❏ Our program provides resources that encourage families to establish a medical home.

- ❏ We offer families information about human services, such as social services, county extension services, and early intervention programs.

- ❏ We offer information about wellness resources, including child dieticians and developmentally appropriate physical activity programs.

- ❏ Our program has contacts with local school districts. We can link families to early childhood services in their school district.

- ❏ Our program has developed contacts with organizations that observe, assess, and intervene for children with suspected or diagnosed special needs or challenging behaviors.

- ❏ We provide families with information about food and nutrition programs, such as WIC.

- ❏ We offer families information about sports, physical activities, and fitness facilities to encourage active lifestyles.

- ❏ We provide families with information about parent and family education resources.

❏ We offer families information about resources that service families in crisis (for example, domestic abuse services, substance abuse services, and family therapy practitioners).

❏ Our program connects families to services available in their primary language.

Did you know? If you are new to the community or are just learning about local early childhood resources, a very good place to begin is your area Child Care Resource and Referral (CCR&R) agency. These operate under a variety of names and offer different programs in different areas. Your licensing representative or your child care health consultant can put you in touch with your local CCR&R.

Decision Making

You make many decisions each day when you work with young children. Your decisions are guided by the mission, policies, and procedures of your program. Families also make many decisions each day that affect the health and well-being of their children. Parents are the primary decision makers on issues affecting their children's health and welfare.

In selecting your program, families have agreed to share some of their decision making with you. As you get to know them, you can incorporate their preferences into your planning and daily decisions about caring for their children. For example, you may have made some decisions about foods served during celebrations in your program based on what you know about nutrition. As you get to know families, you may learn more about their culture and the foods that are used in their family celebrations. This may affect your decisions and possibly alter them.

Many programs invite family members to participate in making some or all of the significant decisions about policies, procedures, philosophy, and mission. These programs engage families fully in governance and share all or most of the decision making with family members.

In most early childhood or child care programs, you balance the interests of several or many families when you need to make decisions. Some families may prefer one course of action; other families may prefer a different one. In some cases, your decisions will be based on regulations or other factors that are not in your control. For example, you cannot decide to continue using old cribs if they no longer meet regulations.

To balance the interests of many families, you must have effective strategies for gathering information, soliciting feedback, and engaging families in decision making. And you need to know when it is appropriate to do so.

DECISION MAKING

Goal: We improve our program's ability to meet children's health, safety, and wellness needs by engaging families in making decisions about the program.

❑ Our annual survey asks about family perceptions of the program's health and wellness strategies. We ask what areas of the program can be improved to meet their needs. Results of the survey are shared with families, and suggestions and improvements are implemented when possible.

❑ A system is in place for families to offer suggestions or make observations about the program. If family members choose to do so, they can offer suggestions anonymously.

Did you know? Consider placing a suggestion box near the area where parents look for information about program events. Some adults prefer to give suggestions anonymously and find suggestion boxes an excellent way to offer new, and often creative, ideas.

❑ Practices are in place so families' concerns and suggestions are acted on in a timely way.

❑ A parent advisory group or other structure exists so families can become more deeply involved in the program's decision making.

❑ Diversity is embraced, respected, and considered in planning family involvement opportunities.

Section 23

Leading Program Staff Members

Program leaders may be called *center directors, executive directors, site supervisors*, or any number of other titles. In family child care programs, they may also function as the teacher. Program leaders are typically responsible for a wide range of duties, including supervision of teachers, assistant teachers, volunteers, and others providing direct care and instruction to children in the program. The work of program leaders directly and indirectly influences the quality of the care and education provided to young children.

One of the most important functions program leaders fulfill is selecting, training, and supervising program staff members. Choosing the adults who will work directly with young children and affect their health and well-being is crucial. One of the reasons program leaders are often mentioned as critical to the quality of early childhood programs is their role in selecting and developing programs' teachers. Gwen Morgan (2000) writes, "The director must achieve quality through the work of others, an often frustrating task that demands skills and knowledge" (42).

You can easily see the link between selecting highly qualified adults to work with young children and quality of care. It is more challenging to understand how much the work environment affects the care adults are able to provide. Paula Jorde Bloom, Ann Hentschel, and Jill Bella (2010) reinforce the importance of the work environment in the overall quality of care provided by a program: "Most of us do not stop to analyze the organizational climate of our workplace, but the climate does influence our behavior, our feelings about our jobs, and how comfortable we feel in expressing our opinions. Without question, the climate of our programs impacts how well we perform our responsibilities and the quality of our day-to-day interactions with children, parents, and co-workers" (Bloom, Hentschel, and Bella, 1).

Organizational climate and work environment are affected by many factors, including how staff members are selected and trained for their jobs, how supervision is conducted, and how staff members can have a say in the way the program is run. The safety of the work environment and the ways that staff members' physical and emotional health are supported influence the organizational climate. Morgan (2010) explains: "The director's decisions on personnel policies, benefits, and work processes are all directly related to the supportive climate of the organization" (43). Directors make decisions about how things get done in the program. These decisions can contribute to safety, or they can create hazards. For example, the director can decide to replace a broken piece of furniture, preventing an injury, or the director can create the budget in a way that allows an adequate number of teachers to safely supervise a field trip.

This section will address:

• Safe and healthy workplace environment: Staff members have a right to expect a safe workplace. Keeping the workplace safe requires a focus on factors in the environment that help adults remain safe, and policies and procedures that focus on staff members.

- Physical health of teachers: Physically healthy teachers can provide better care for young children. Teachers and other staff members must be healthy so they do not transmit illnesses to children in care.

- Stress and resilience: Caring for children can be a stressful job. Leaders can implement policies and practices that help to reduce stress and provide opportunities for relief when stress becomes overwhelming.

- Decision making and involvement: Many decisions are made in child care programs each day. Involving staff members and others in decision making can contribute to a positive work environment.

- Recruitment and selection: Selecting caring adults to work with young children is an important responsibility of program leaders.

- Supervision and training: Caring for young children requires training and ongoing professional development. Leaders provide the environment in which training takes place and routine supervision to ensure that policies and practices are implemented as intended.

Safe and Healthy Workplace Environment

Although the primary purpose of early childhood programs is safe and healthy care of children, they must also provide safe and healthy environments for staff members. Like children, you and the other adults in your program can do your best only in an environment where you are free from physical risks and likely to remain healthy.

Child care facilities are designed to protect the health and safety of young children, so they are usually very safe work environments. But a number of hazards can affect you and other adults working in the program. Common hazards in child care programs include lifting and slipping and falling on uneven or wet floors.

Some hazards in child care programs are hazards you could encounter in any workplace or home. But some hazards are unique to the work you do with young children. For example, exposure to children's body fluids poses hazards. You need to take precautions when changing diapers, administering first aid, and performing other tasks that bring you into contact with urine, feces, mucous, blood, and other fluids.

Your program may store and use chemicals that are potentially hazardous. For example, you may have disinfectants or **pesticides** stored at your facility. The U.S. Occupational Safety and Health Administration (OSHA) issues regulations that help you and other staff members have a safe workplace. OSHA requires that employees be made aware of potential hazards from chemicals (for example, pesticides and cleaning agents) in the workplace.

SAFE AND HEALTHY WORKPLACE ENVIRONMENT

Goal: Our program maintains an environment that is safe and healthy for staff members and volunteers.

❑ Our facility and grounds are inspected at least weekly for hazards that could hurt staff members.

❑ Staff members and volunteers are trained in safe use of program equipment, such as **fire extinguishers**, copy machines, and kitchen appliances.

❑ Our program provides safety data sheets for all potentially hazardous products used in cleaning, pest control, and other maintenance.

❑ Staff members and volunteers are trained about risks associated with chemicals used or stored in the facility.

❑ Staff members and volunteers receive training about risks from exposure to body fluids.

❑ Supplies like nonlatex gloves are readily available to encourage the use of **standard precautions**. Standard precautions lower risks to teachers from contact with body fluids and blood.

❑ Female staff members and volunteers of childbearing age are trained about the risks of cytomegalovirus (CMV). Hygiene procedures, such as hand washing, are taught to minimize risks.

❑ We post **evacuation** plans in each area of the facility, including areas used only by staff members. Exits are clearly marked.

❑ Staff members are encouraged to interact with the program's child care health consultant and to ask about workplace safety.

❑ Signs are used to warn staff members about spills, wet floors, and other potential slip, trip, or fall hazards.

❑ Materials used frequently by staff members are stored in easy-to-reach areas. Doing so reduces the risk of ladders and step stools.

Following safety practices also ensures you are a good role model for children. If you stand on a chair or shelf to reach something up high, then it is likely a child will try to mimic your actions and put himself in danger. Teach children by modeling safety in all situations.

❑ Hot surfaces or hot containers are labeled. Protective equipment, such as hot pads and gloves, is provided.

❑ Children over thirty pounds use steps to reach changing tables. This eliminates or minimizes the need for teachers to lift heavy children frequently.

❑ Workers' compensation or a disability plan is in place for when work-related injuries occur. Staff members are aware of the plan.

❑ Records of all adult injuries are maintained and reviewed annually. Actions are taken to prevent similar injuries in the future.

Did you know? Reducing back injuries is a very effective way to help teachers remain safe and healthy. Lifting children is a normal and expected part of your job. Learning safe lifting techniques is one way to protect your health. Your child care health consultant can provide information about safe lifting. *Safe Lifting Techniques of Children* is an excellent informative brochure created by the Occupational Health Clinics for Ontario Workers. Find it online at http://www.ohcow.on.ca/resources/handbooks/childlift/safeliftingbrochure.pdf.

Physical Health of Teachers

You and the other teachers in your program must be physically well to care for young children. Physical health is important to prevent transmitting of illness to the children in your care. Your health is also important to providing the level of care that children require. When you are ill, you cannot be as active as you need to be. You do not have enough stamina to keep up with active young children. You may miss important supervisory details that could endanger children. You and the other adults in your early childhood program are role models for young children. Taking precautions needed to prevent or minimize illness subtly teaches them important life lessons about health and wellness.

Balancing the sometimes competing needs of teachers, children, and families is a challenge for every program. Sometimes you're tempted to continue working when you are feeling ill because of your dedication to the children. You know that parents count on you to be available every day and that it is hard for them and the children when you are absent. But it is important for you and your program leadership to develop policies and systems that allow you to address your own health needs without putting the children at risk or causing undue hardships on families. If you are a family child care provider or work alone with children each day, finding time to recuperate away from the children can be particularly difficult. Identifying potential substitutes that you can call on when you are sick is an essential precaution.

PHYSICAL HEALTH OF TEACHERS

Goal: Our program's policies and practices encourage teachers' physical health.

❏ Teachers are required to have routine physical examinations at least once each year. Documentation is provided to the program.

❏ Teachers are required to have up-to-date **immunizations** before working with young children.

❏ Our employee policies clearly exclude teachers who show signs of illness from working with children.

❏ Program leaders conduct daily checks of teachers to be sure no signs of illness are present.

❏ Teachers who become ill during the workday are immediately separated from the children.

❏ Our employee policies clearly describe how teachers should notify the program when they are ill and how to arrange for substitutes.

❏ Staff members' benefits include paid sick days so staff members are not penalized for illness.

❏ Qualified substitutes are readily available so ill teachers are not required to work with children. Adequate adult-to-child **ratios** are maintained.

❏ Staff members have health care benefits so they can seek medical treatment when they become ill. They can obtain preventive care to minimize illness.

❏ Staff members' benefits include access to programs that support healthy lifestyles (for example, health club membership, smoking cessation programs, diet and nutrition counseling).

❏ Families are notified when a teacher is diagnosed with a communicable illness.

❏ Staff members are provided with educational materials that encourage healthy lifestyles.

❏ Staff meetings, trainings, and other gatherings model healthy habits by including healthy foods and emphasizing health and wellness.

❏ The workplace environment is kept clean to prevent illness among staff members.

Did you know? How did you sleep last night? Getting seven to eight hours of rest each night is an important healthy habit you can embrace to protect your health and safety. Getting enough sleep means you are always well rested, recharged, and ready for a full day of active play with children. When you are well rested, you are also more attentive. Being well rested helps your body fight off illnesses, so you are less likely to become sick.

Stress and Resilience

You probably chose early childhood education because you enjoy working with young children. You find the work satisfying. But even the most dedicated professionals have days when the challenges of caring for children are emotionally draining and affect their work. Although catering to the needs of young children can be stressful, you can't allow those stresses to endanger the children.

Everyone encounters stress. Most of the time, you can manage that stress successfully. You may be running late, thinking of an upcoming event that requires hard work, or fretting about some bills you need to pay. Most of the time, you can respond to these everyday stresses easily, without diverting your attention from the care of the children. Sometimes the stresses in your life are too big or too numerous to manage easily. When you are under a great deal of stress or unable to effectively manage it, you may make poor decisions, become harsh with the children, or fail to notice important things that put children in harm's way. Program leadership can help you minimize the impact of stress and protect children from the risks associated with your stress.

One of the most effective methods of reducing stress and its impact is to ensure that the program's policies, practices, and environment support teachers' resilience. Similar to those of children, resilience skills can be either nurtured or diminished based on the daily experiences and life events a person encounters. While programs and administration are not responsible for developing competencies in adults the same way they are for children, it is in the best interest of all to support resilience in teachers. In essence, teachers themselves are their most important teaching tool, and they must care for themselves as a musician would care for her instrument or a carpenter would care for his tools.

STRESS AND RESILIENCE

Goal: Our program's policies and practices minimize stressors, help teachers to manage stress, and reinforce resilience.

❑ Teachers have regular breaks away from the children. The breaks are scheduled at least once every four hours.

❑ Teachers receive training that helps them to recognize signs of stress in themselves or others that could result in injuries to children.

❑ Work schedules are planned so teachers do not work more than eight hours a day or more than forty hours a week.

❑ Substitutes are available so teachers can take days off for personal reasons or for vacation.

❑ Our facility has a place for teachers to take breaks and plan away from the children.

❑ Program leaders conduct regular observations of teachers, provide feedback on performance, and detect any concerns about teacher performance.

❑ A grievance procedure is in place to negotiate differences among staff members.

❑ Staff members have access to resources and training opportunities to help them improve their knowledge and skills.

❑ Teachers have access to resources that address stresses in their personal or professional lives.

❑ There are regular opportunities to share teaching challenges with one another, collaborate, and jointly solve problems.

❑ Staff members' activities and meetings include fun and relaxing exercises.

❑ Staff members' retreats are held, preferably off-site, to renew energy and provide new knowledge.

❑ Funding is set aside when possible for staff members to participate in professional development activities.

❑ Leaders share difficult news or changes honestly and positively.

❑ Gossip is not tolerated in our program.

❑ All staff members' information, both professional and personal, is treated confidentially.

Did you know? In a program where you spend day in and day out with the same people, it seems inevitable that gossip and conflict will arise. It is tempting to blow off a bit of steam by expressing your frustration about a coworker or parent. But allowing this, even once, will affect the tone of the whole program. Of course, it is natural to discuss frustrations, but problem resolution should be the objective of all communication regarding conflict. This is especially important for leaders, who set the tone for everyone else.

❑ Conflict between teachers is resolved professionally and immediately.

❑ Teachers have some control over their daily work.

❑ Teachers' input is valued.

Decision Making and Involvement

The old adage "Two heads are better than one" has remained good advice for centuries because it summarizes what we know: adults can work together to make good things happen. People in any work environment appreciate having a voice in the way things get done. Many points of view usually produce better decisions for the entire program. Paula Jorde Bloom's (2010) research on early childhood work environments describes the importance of including teachers in program decision making: "In general, when teachers feel that their program's decision-making structure is fair and values their input, they are more likely to make a commitment to program goals. Centers with positive organizational climates encourage staff to take an active role in centerwide decision making. Research suggests that staff participation in making decisions also has positive impact on the level of job satisfaction they experience" (Bloom, Hentschel, and Bella, 14).

Certainly some decisions must be made by your program's leaders, owners, or governing boards. But many decisions benefit from the input of the teachers who work most closely with children and their families. Not every program decision needs to be put to a vote. You and other staff members can be involved in decision making by building consensus or voting.

DECISION MAKING AND INVOLVEMENT

Goal: We create a healthy environment by encouraging all adults working in the program to provide input in decisions that guide the program.

❑ Our annual survey of staff members asks their perceptions of the program's health and wellness strategies and where the program could better meet their needs.

❑ A system is in place for staff members to offer suggestions or make observations about the program. If staff members choose to do so, they can offer suggestions anonymously.

Did you know? A suggestion box is a simple tool to gather suggestions from staff members in the program. Place it in an accessible area. Allow staff members to offer suggestions anonymously if they want to.

❑ Staff meetings or other structures, such as advisory councils or program operating committees, allow teachers to become more deeply involved in the program's decision making through discussion, goal setting, and strategic planning.

❑ Our complaint procedure explains how issues can be solved jointly by teachers and the administrators.

Recruitment and Selection

High-quality care depends on the staff members in programs for children. Many adults find the idea of working with children intriguing, but not every adult interested in a caregiving role is suited to work in child care programs. Selecting teachers to work with young children is a significant responsibility.

You and all of the adults who work in the program must meet the qualifications of licensing agencies to work in child care programs. Merely identifying those who meet the licensing agencies' qualifications does not constitute acceptable screening. Such qualifications are minimum expectations. Meeting only these standards does not ensure that your program has people with the skills and knowledge needed to provide high-quality care and education. Professional organizations like the National Association for the Education of Young Children (NAEYC) and the National Association of Child Care Professionals (NACCP) have set guidelines for professionals working with young children. These guidelines typically demand a higher standard than licensing requirements. They provide a good starting point for determining qualifications. Your state may also have a quality rating and improvement system that defines the enhanced staff member qualifications associated with higher levels of quality.

Leaders selecting staff members to work in child care programs are looking for candidates who can model a healthy lifestyle, are emotionally well and show resilience to stress, are committed to ongoing education and performance improvement, and will work alongside others congenially.

RECRUITMENT AND SELECTION

Goal: We support children's healthy development by selecting highly qualified adults to work in the program.

❑ Our open positions are advertised in several publications and venues to attract a diverse candidate pool.

❑ We emphasize hiring teachers who reflect the population served by the program.

❑ We emphasize hiring teachers who speak the languages spoken by families in the program.

❑ The program has and follows a policy of nondiscrimination in hiring. It complies with state and federal regulations.

❑ Applicants are given every protection under the Americans with Disabilities Act (ADA). Reasonable accommodations are made so applicants receive equal opportunities to apply and be hired for jobs.

Did you know? Your program must comply with the requirements of the Americans with Disabilities Act (ADA) in its hiring practices. For more information about these practices, consult *Job Accommodation Network* online at http://askjan.org. This website provides information about workplace accommodations and the ADA. You can also use it to submit questions to experts.

❑ Our program hires only candidates who can demonstrate that they meet the legally required qualifications for the available positions. These may include citizenship or legal residency.

❑ All teachers hired for assisting positions are at least eighteen years old and have a high school diploma or the equivalent and on-the-job training.

❑ All teachers hired for lead positions are at least twenty-one years old and have a bachelor's degree related to child development or early childhood education, at least one year of experience, and participate in on-the-job training.

❑ All candidates are subject to a background check, including fingerprinting.

❑ All candidates provide at least three professional references, including at least one reference who has observed the candidate with children. All references are contacted before a candidate is hired, and reference information is documented.

Did you know? Interviewing and checking references are important tasks, but many child care leaders don't have resources to guide them through these important processes. In fact, there are legal guidelines about what you can and can't ask. It is important to ask open-ended questions, ask questions about educational and child guidance philosophies, and, most important, listen more than you talk. And be sure interviews and references are documented.

❑ All candidates provide their employment history. Previous employers are asked about the candidate's punctuality, dependability, and overall work habits.

❑ All candidates participate in at least one face-to-face interview before hire. During the interview, they are asked to discuss their philosophy of education and to respond to situation-based questions.

❑ All candidates have the opportunity to observe in the classroom before accepting a position.

❑ When allowed by law, candidates under close supervision spend time in the classroom conducting an activity or interactions with children before being hired.

❑ Experienced lead teachers are offered the chance to participate in interviews and to provide feedback about candidates.

❑ Managers responsible for hiring teachers have been trained in interview techniques and the legal requirements associated with hiring.

❑ Outreach is made to all ethnic communities served by the program.

Supervision and Training

In most states, adults qualify to work in child care programs based on their age, education, and work experience. Many licensing regulations set minimum age requirements for adults working with young children in child care or early childhood programs. Typically, adults can qualify to work in assisting roles (aides, assistant teachers, helpers) with little or no education or experience. Adults working in roles of greater responsibility (teachers, lead teachers, directors) usually need to have at least some education beyond high school. In some cases, they need experience working in assisting roles.

Pre-service training requirements (those that teachers must have before working with young children), vary from state to state. Once candidates are hired, they typically participate in some kind of **orientation**. Orientation training is designed to introduce new employees to the program's policies, procedures, and operating norms. Pre-service requirements and orientation requirements often overlap or are used interchangeably in licensing regulations. Some states have extensive orientation requirements for those who work with young children. Other states have none. Regardless of state requirements, programs can set pre-service and orientation training requirements that exceed those of the state licensing agency.

To continue growing and developing as a professional, you should participate in continuing education, also called **in-service training**. Licensing requirements may state the topics and number of hours of in-service training required each year. All teachers should meet the licensing requirements for in-service training, as well as the following recommendations.

PRE-SERVICE TRAINING

Goal: The health and well-being of children in our program is protected by ensuring that teachers have extensive training before they work with children.

❑ Teachers are trained in first aid before working with children.

❑ Teachers are certified in **cardiopulmonary resuscitation** (CPR) before working with children.

❑ Teachers are trained in child development, including the following:
  ❑ developmental stages
  ❑ positive ways to support cognitive, social-emotional, and physical development
  ❑ appropriate guidance and **discipline**
  ❑ diversity and acceptance of cultural differences
  ❑ developing and implementing plans for children with varying needs

❑ Teachers receive health and safety training, including the following:
  ❑ procedures for preventing the spread of illness, such as hand washing, diapering, and food handling
  ❑ procedures for identifying common illnesses
  ❑ procedures for group medication
  ❑ policies and practices on nutrition and eating

❑ If infants are cared for in the program, teachers receive training that includes the following:
  ❑ safe sleep practices that reduce the risk of SIDS
  ❑ practices to calm crying infants, information about the risks associated with **shaken baby syndrome**, and ways to identify children who may be victims of shaken baby syndrome

❑ Teachers are trained to prepare for emergencies, including the following:
  ❑ basic first aid training and infant/child CPR certification
  ❑ responses and drills for weather and natural disaster emergencies

❑ Teachers are trained to recognize and report child abuse.

❑ Pre-service training is documented in each employee's file.

Did you know? Some employers require candidates to complete their pre-service training before they are hired. For example, a program may require that all employees complete a credential or a degree program, including all of the desired pre-service requirements. Other programs provide training to new employees to help them meet pre-service requirements.

ORIENTATION TO THE PROGRAM

Goal: We protect the health and well-being of children in our program by orienting all staff members before they work with children.

❑ All staff members, regardless of position, participate in an extensive orientation to the program.

❑ Staff members receive information about the program's mission and philosophy.

❑ Staff members are oriented to the program's emphasis on child wellness.

❑ Staff members receive orientation information stressing their role as models for children's behavior and healthy lifestyle.

❑ Staff members receive written copies of all program policies. Managers share the policies with new employees.

❑ Staff members receive orientation to the resources available to the program: child care health consultant, licensing agent, and others used by or available to the program.

❑ Staff members are oriented to the occupational risks of handling body fluids.

❑ Teachers are introduced to the group of children they will work with and receive information about children's allergies, illnesses, and special needs.

❑ Teachers learn about the guidance policy and procedures for child guidance used in the program.

❑ During orientation, teachers are given opportunities to ask questions and to receive thorough answers.

❑ Teachers are given written copies of staff policies, such as a staff handbook, during orientation. They have opportunities to read the policies and ask questions. Staff members indicate in writing that they have read and understood the policies.

❑ Orientation training is documented in each employee's file.

Did you know? Orientation is a great time for new employees to learn about the policies, producers, and inner workings of a program. It is also a great time to build teamwork and to help new employees feel connected to others in the program. To help this connection form, you might appoint a buddy for each new staff member. The buddy's job is to provide camaraderie, introduce the new employee to the team, and provide the beginning of a support network.

ONGOING TRAINING OR IN-SERVICE TRAINING

Goal: We support children's healthy development by providing ongoing training that enhances knowledge and skills of staff members.

❑ All staff members, regardless of position, participate in ongoing education or in-service training.

❑ Teachers participate in at least thirty clock hours of training each year.

❑ In-service training focuses on the training needs of staff members. Training choices are based on needs rather than wants. They match the skill and knowledge needs identified in performance evaluations.

❑ In-service training is conducted by highly qualified trainers with subject-matter expertise. They are skilled in adult learning practices.

❑ Staff members who handle food receive ongoing training in food safety and nutrition.

❑ Teachers receive ongoing training about the age group of children with whom they work.

❑ Staff members receive ongoing training to promote cultural competence and relationship building with family members.

❑ Staff members receive ongoing training that emphasizes community resources that can benefit children, families, and teachers.

SUPERVISION

Goal: We support children's healthy development by supervising the work of all staff members.

❑ Program leaders schedule time each day to observe teachers at work.

❑ Program leaders share their observations with teachers.

❑ Program leaders and teachers develop goals for improvement based on observations of the teachers' work.

❑ Staff members participate in formal performance evaluations at least once annually.

❑ Staff members are encouraged to provide feedback on their own performance as part of performance evaluations.

❑ Program leaders and teachers create professional development plans each year based on performance, training needs, and interests of teachers.

❑ Program leaders are trained to observe the performance of staff members, evaluate job performance, and provide feedback.

Section 24

Facility and Financial Management

Managing the facility and the financial aspects of the program has a big impact on your ability to meet the health and safety needs of children. You may not immediately see the connection between hiring a vendor or creating a budget and children's safety, but a connection does exist. Most decisions made in child care programs affect children's well-being. For example, hiring a contractor to maintain the air-conditioning system may not seem to have a direct impact on children. But the choice of a highly qualified contractor may determine the program's air quality, the health of the children and adults in the building, and the atmosphere in which children receive care.

Managing a facility in which child care or early education is provided can be complex. You may have little knowledge of heating systems, air conditioning, or building maintenance, but you find yourself responsible for these systems. Most program leaders use vendors or contractors to provide services in areas where they are not experts.

Vendors are people or organizations that provide products or services to the program for a fee. Most child care programs use a wide variety of vendors. Programs may also use contracted services, such as a lawn care service, to maintain the building or the grounds. These vendors are contracted to provide specific ongoing services needed by the program.

You can provide for children's health and safety only if you have made adequate financial provisions. Many of the policies, procedures, and activities that help ensure children's health and safety have a financial impact on your program. For example, providing first aid training to staff members usually costs something. Your program may pay for the training itself and perhaps for the staff members' time to complete the training. These costs must be included in your program's budget so funds are available when the expenses arise. Similarly, if you are planning to use contracts or vendors to provide services to maintain your facility, you must budget to ensure that they can be paid. Your careful financial planning protects your investment in solid policies and procedures.

This section will address:

- Vendors and contracted services: Many programs use contracted services or vendors to deliver supplies or to perform duties such as landscaping or waste removal or to offer enrichment classes. These people can contribute to the safety of the program but must be selected and supervised carefully.

- Financial planning: Operating a child care program requires careful planning for expenses that contribute to the health and safety of the program. For example, adequate funds must be available to purchase safe materials and to maintain the facility.

Vendors and Contracted Services

The health and safety of the children and adults in your program depend on a safe, healthy environment. You can do a lot to maintain the environment yourself, but you seldom have the time or expertise to address all of the facility's needs. Moreover, there may be services or opportunities you want to offer to children and families that you do not have the ability or expertise to offer without the support of a vendor.

Maintaining a home or a commercial building is specialized work. It should be done by professionals who are trained, and in some cases certified, in specific skills. Doing your own construction or maintenance work may appear to save money, but it could be dangerous if you do not have a thorough knowledge of codes and mechanical systems. Facility vendors or contracted services used in child care programs include cleaning services, heating, ventilation, and air conditioning (HVAC) services, plumbing, general maintenance, and landscaping services. Your program may employ services as needed, or you may have ongoing contracts for routine inspections and repairs. If your program is part of a larger organization or complex, you may have access to on-site staff members who perform facility services.

Many child care programs also contract with vendors to offer enrichment classes for children, such as dance or soccer. Even though these vendors have more experience working with children, they still need careful attention and supervision to be sure they are safe.

FACILITY VENDORS AND CONTRACTED SERVICES

Goal: We use vendors and contract services to protect the health and safety of children.

- ❏ Highly qualified vendors are contracted to maintain the building's systems, for example, heating, cooling, and water.

- ❏ Vendors are aware of the licensing guidelines that govern our program.

- ❏ Vendors are experienced in working with facilities for children.

- ❏ Vendors are aware of the potential risks to young children posed by building systems such as heating and air-conditioning or materials used to maintain the systems.

- ❏ Vendors use only products considered safe for use around children.

- ❏ Vendors visiting the facility are never left alone in areas where children are present.

- ❏ Whenever possible, vendors complete facility work during hours when children are not present.

❑ When work must be conducted during hours of operation, children are cared for away from work areas.

❑ Vendors who have regular access to the facility when children are present, such as cleaning or maintenance workers, have background clearances to ensure that they have no history of child abuse.

PROGRAM VENDORS OR CONTRACTED SERVICES

Goal: We ensure that vendors or contractors working directly with children provide safe and appropriate experiences.

❑ We have a legal contract with vendors that includes proof of their insurance.

❑ We ensure vendors have a background check that includes a comprehensive background check.

❑ We ask vendors for references before they work in our program.

❑ We do not count vendors in our adult-to-child ratio and continue to supervise children even when engaged in an activity with a vendor.

❑ Vendors are not left alone with children.

❑ We assess vendors' programming on a regular basis to be sure it is developmentally appropriate.

❑ We monitor vendors' communication with parents and families.

❑ Vendors must never punish or **discipline** children.

Financial Planning

Program leaders are responsible for the financial health of the program. Your program may be a family child care home or a large commercial child care center. Either way, you will need a budget that projects the program's expected income and the expenses it is likely to incur.

You must budget to reflect the mission and goals of the program. Your budget should include funds for the health and safety activities described in earlier sections of this book. Without adequate funds, you cannot implement many of the plans you have made or sustain health and safety programs you have already put in place.

Your budget will address many facets of your overall program. For example, you will budget for program supplies, such as crayons, paints, and books. You will budget for staff members' wages and benefits. The items in the following checklist reflect health and safety activities or requirements that should be included in your program budget.

FINANCIAL PLANNING

Goal: The finances of our program are managed so sufficient resources are available to promote children's health and safety.

❑ Program leaders develop a budget for the program each year. The budget is approved by the program's governing boards or other program leaders.

❑ The budget provides adequate wages for teachers to minimize turnover.

❑ The program budget includes funds for training and professional development of staff members.

❑ The program budget allows teachers to take breaks, plan, and do other preparation work away from the children.

❑ The program budget includes funds for substitutes when teachers are ill.

❑ The program budget funds the purchase of equipment to replace items that are worn, damaged, or recalled.

❑ The program budget provides sufficient funds so fresh foods can be purchased for meals and snacks.

❑ The program budget provides sufficient funds so the facility can be regularly cleaned.

❑ The program budget provides sufficient funds for contracted services by a highly qualified child care health consultant.

❑ The program budget provides funds for replacing or supplementing cushioning materials around climbing equipment.

❑ The program budget is audited by an external auditor each year.

Appendixes

Action Plan

Part: _____

Section: _____

Goal: _____

Indicator/Page Number	Action Steps	Resources	Responsible Party	Timeline	Cost	Notes	Success!

Indicator/Page Number	Action Steps	Resources	Responsible Party	Timeline	Cost	Notes	Success!

Active Start: A Statement of Physical Activity Guidelines for Children from Birth to Age 5

Guidelines

Guidelines for Infants:

Guideline 1.   Infants should interact with caregivers in daily physical activities that are dedicated to exploring movement and the environment.

Guideline 2.   Caregivers should place infants in settings that encourage and stimulate movement experiences and active play for short periods of time several times a day.

Guideline 3.   Infants' physical activity should promote skill development in movement.

Guideline 4.   Infants should be placed in an environment that meets or exceeds recommended safety standards for performing large-muscle activities.

Guideline 5.   Those in charge of infants' well-being are responsible for understanding the importance of physical activity and should promote movement skills by providing opportunities for structured and unstructured physical activity.

Guidelines for Toddlers:

Guideline 1.   Toddlers should engage in a total of at least 30 minutes of structured physical activity each day.

Guideline 2.   Toddlers should engage in at least 60 minutes—and up to several hours—per day of unstructured physical activity and should not be sedentary for more than 60 minutes at a time, except when sleeping.

Guideline 3. Toddlers should be given ample opportunities to develop movement skills that will serve as the building blocks for future motor skillfulness and physical activity.

Guideline 4. Toddlers should have access to indoor and outdoor areas that meet or exceed recommended safety standards for performing large-muscle activities.

Guideline 5. Those in charge of toddlers' well-being are responsible for understanding the importance of physical activity and promoting movement skills by providing opportunities for structured and unstructured physical activity and movement experiences.

Guidelines for Preschoolers:

Guideline 1. Preschoolers should accumulate at least 60 minutes of structured physical activity each day.

Guideline 2. Preschoolers should engage in at least 60 minutes—and up to several hours—of unstructured physical activity each day, and should not be sedentary for more than 60 minutes at a time, except when sleeping.

Guideline 3. Preschoolers should be encouraged to develop competence in fundamental motor skills that will serve as the building blocks for future motor skillfulness and physical activity.

Guideline 4. Preschoolers should have access to indoor and outdoor areas that meet or exceed recommended safety standards for performing large-muscle activities.

Guideline 5. Caregivers and parents in charge of preschoolers' health and well-being are responsible for understanding the importance of physical activity and for promoting movement skills by providing opportunities for structured and unstructured physical activity.

Reprinted from *Active Start: A Statement of Physical Activity Guidelines for Children from Birth to Age 5* with permission from the National Association for Sport and Physical Education (NASPE), 1900 Association Drive, Reston, VA 20191, www.NASPEinfo.org.

STANDARD 3.2.1.4: Diaper Changing Procedure

The following diaper-changing procedure should be posted in the changing area, should be followed for all diaper changes, and should be used as part of staff evaluation of caregivers/teachers who diaper. The signage should be simple and should be in multiple languages if caregivers/teachers who speak multiple languages are involved in diapering. All employees who will diaper should undergo training and periodic assessment of diapering practices. Caregivers/teachers should never leave a child unattended on a table or countertop, even for an instant. A safety strap or harness should not be used on the diaper-changing table. If an emergency arises, caregivers/teachers should bring any child on an elevated surface to the floor or take the child with them.

An EPA-registered disinfectant suitable for the surface material that is being disinfected should be used. If an EPA-registered product is not available, then household bleach diluted with water is a practical alternative. All cleaning and disinfecting solutions should be stored to be accessible to the caregiver/teacher but out of reach of any child.

Step 1: Get organized. Before bringing the child to the diaper-changing area, perform hand hygiene, gather and bring supplies to the diaper-changing area:

a. Nonabsorbent paper liner large enough to cover the changing surface from the child's shoulders to beyond the child's feet;

b. Unused diaper, clean clothes (if you need them);

c. Wipes for cleaning the child's genitalia and buttocks removed from the container or dispensed so the container will not be touched during diaper changing;

d. A wet cloth or paper towel;

e. A plastic bag for any soiled clothes or cloth diapers;

f. Disposable gloves, if you plan to use them (put gloves on before handling soiled clothing or diapers) and remove them before handling clean diapers and clothing;

g. A thick application of any diaper cream (e.g., zinc oxide ointment), when appropriate, removed from the container to a piece of disposable material such as facial or toilet tissue.

Step 2: Carry the child to the changing table, keeping soiled clothing away from you and any surfaces you cannot easily clean and sanitize after the change.

a. Always keep a hand on the child;

b. If the child's feet cannot be kept out of the diaper or from contact with soiled skin during the changing process, remove the child's shoes and socks so the child does not contaminate these surfaces with stool or urine during the diaper changing.

Step 3: Clean the child's diaper area.

   a. Place the child on the diaper change surface and unfasten the diaper, but leave the soiled diaper under the child;

   b. If safety pins are used, close each pin immediately once it is removed and keep pins out of the child's reach (never hold pins in your mouth);

   c. Lift the child's legs as needed to use disposable wipes to clean the skin on the child's genitalia and buttocks and prevent recontamination from a soiled diaper. If there is a need to clean between the labia of an infant girl, use only a wet cloth or paper towel. Remove stool and urine from front to back and use a fresh wipe each time you swipe. Put the soiled wipes into the soiled diaper or directly into a plastic-lined, hands-free covered can.

Step 4: Remove the soiled diaper and clothing without contaminating any surface not already in contact with stool or urine.

   a. Fold the soiled surface of the diaper inward;

   b. Put soiled disposable diapers in a covered, plastic-lined, hands-free covered can. If reusable cloth diapers are used, put the soiled cloth diaper and its contents (without emptying or rinsing) in a plastic bag or into a plastic-lined, hands-free covered can to give to parents/ guardians or laundry service;

   c. Put soiled clothes in a plastic-lined, hands-free plastic bag;

   d. If gloves were used, remove them using the proper technique and put them into a plastic-lined, hands-free covered can;

   e. Whether or not gloves were used, use a disposable antibacterial wipe or alcohol-based hand sanitizer to clean the surfaces of the caregiver/teacher's hands and an application to clean the child's hands, and put the wipes, if used, into the plastic-lined, hands-free covered can. Allow sanitized hands to dry completely before proceeding;

   f. Check for spills under the child. If there are any, use the paper that extends under the child's feet to fold over the soiled area so a fresh, unsoiled paper surface is now under the child's buttocks.

Step 5: Put on a clean diaper and dress the child.

   a. Slide a fresh diaper under the child;

   b. Use a facial or toilet tissue or wear clean disposable gloves to apply any necessary diaper creams, discarding the tissue or glove in a covered, plastic-lined, hands-free covered can;

   c. Note and plan to report any skin problems such as redness, skin cracks, or bleeding;

   d. Fasten the diaper; if pins are used, place your hand between the child and the diaper when inserting the pin.

Step 6: Wash the child's hands and return the child to a supervised area.

    a. Use soap and warm water, between 60°F and 120°F, at a sink to wash the child's hands, if you can.

Step 7: Clean and disinfect the diaper-changing surface.

    a. Dispose of the disposable paper liner used on the diaper-changing surface in a plastic-lined, hands-free covered can;

    b. If clothing was soiled, securely tie the plastic bag used to store the clothing and send home;

    c. Remove any visible soil from the changing surface with a disposable paper towel saturated with water and detergent, rinse;

    d. Wet the entire changing surface with a disinfectant that is appropriate for the surface material you are treating. Follow the manufacturer's instructions for use;

    e. Put away the disinfectant. Some types of disinfectants may require rinsing the changing table surface with fresh water afterwards.

Step 8: Perform hand hygiene according to the procedure in Standard 3.2.2.2 and record the diaper change in the child's daily log.

    a. In the daily log, record what was in the diaper and any problems (such as a loose stool, an unusual odor, blood in the stool, or any skin irritation), and report as necessary (2).

RATIONALE:

The procedure for diaper changing is designed to reduce the contamination of surfaces that will later come in contact with uncontaminated surfaces such as hands, furnishings, and floors (1, 3). Posting the multistep procedure may help caregivers/teachers maintain the routine.

Assembling all necessary supplies before bringing the child to the changing area will ensure the child's safety, make the change more efficient, and reduce opportunities for contamination. Taking the supplies out of their containers and leaving the containers in their storage places reduces the likelihood that the storage containers will become contaminated during diaper changing.

Commonly, caregivers/teachers do not use disposable paper that is large enough to cover the area likely to be contaminated during diaper changing. If the paper is large enough, there will be less need to remove visible soil from surfaces later, and there will be enough paper to fold up so the soiled surface is not in contact with clean surfaces while dressing the child.

If the child's foot coverings are not removed during diaper changing and the child kicks during the diaper changing procedure, the foot coverings can become contaminated and subsequently spread contamination throughout the child care area.

If the child's clean buttocks are put down on a soiled surface, the child's skin can be resoiled.

Children's hands often stray into the diaper area (the area of the child's body covered by the diaper) during the diapering process and can then transfer fecal organisms to the environment.

Washing the child's hands will reduce the number of organisms carried into the environment in this way. Infectious organisms are present on the skin and diaper even though they are not seen. To reduce the contamination of clean surfaces, caregiver/teachers should use an antibacterial wipe or alcohol-based hand sanitizer to wipe their hands after removing the gloves, or, if no gloves were used, before proceeding to handle the clean diaper and the clothing.

Some states and credentialing organizations may recommend wearing gloves for diaper changing. Although gloves may not be required, they may provide a barrier against surface contamination of a caregiver/teacher's hands. This may reduce the presence of enteric pathogens under the fingernails and on hand surfaces. Even if gloves are used, caregivers/teachers must perform hand hygiene after each child's diaper changing to prevent the spread of disease-causing agents. To achieve maximum benefit from use of gloves, the caregiver/teacher must remove the gloves properly after cleaning the child's genitalia and buttocks and removing the soiled diaper. Otherwise, retained contaminated gloves could transfer organisms to clean surfaces. Note that sensitivity to latex is a growing problem. If caregivers/teachers or children who are sensitive to latex are present in the facility, non-latex gloves should be used.

A safety strap cannot be relied upon to restrain the child and could become contaminated during diaper changing. Cleaning and disinfecting a strap would be required after every diaper change. Therefore safety straps on diaper-changing surfaces are not recommended.

Prior to disinfecting the changing table, clean any visible soil from the surface with a detergent and rinse well with water. Always follow the manufacturer's instructions for use, application, and storage. If the disinfectant is applied using a spray bottle, always assume that the outside of the spray bottle could be contaminated. Therefore, the spray bottle should be put away before hand hygiene is performed (the last and essential part of every diaper change) (4).

Diaper-changing areas should never be located in food preparation areas and should never be used for temporary placement of food, drinks, or eating utensils.

If parents use the diaper-changing area, they should be required to follow the same diaper changing procedure to minimize contamination of the diaper-changing area and child care.

REFERENCES:

1. Pickering, L. K., C. J. Baker, D. W. Kimberlin, and S. S. Long, eds. 2009. Red book 2009: *Report of the Committee on Infectious Diseases*, 28th ed. Elk Grove Village, IL: American Academy of Pediatrics.

2. National Association for the Education of Young Children. 2007. *Keeping Healthy: Parents, Teachers, and Children*, rev. ed. Washington, DC: NAEYC.

3. Fiene, R. 2002. 13 indicators of quality child care: Research update. Washington, DC: U.S. Department of Health and Human Services, Office of the Assistant Secretary for Planning and Evaluation. http://aspe.hhs.gov/hsp/ccquality-ind02/.

4. North Carolina Child Care Health and Safety Resource Center. Diapering-procedure poster. http://www.healthychildcarenc.org/PDFs/diaper_procedure_english.pdf.

STANDARD 3.2.2.2: Handwashing Procedure

Children and staff members should wash their hands using the following method:

a. Check to be sure a clean, disposable paper (or single-use cloth) towel is available;

b. Turn on warm water, between 60°F and 120°F, to a comfortable temperature;

c. Moisten hands with water and apply soap (not antibacterial) to hands;

d. Rub hands together vigorously until a soapy lather appears, hands are out of the water stream, and continue for at least twenty seconds (sing "Happy Birthday" silently twice) (2). Rub areas between fingers, around nailbeds, under fingernails, jewelry, and back of hands. Nails should be kept short; acrylic nails should not be worn (3);

e. Rinse hands under running water, between 60°F and 120°F, until they are free of soap and dirt. Leave the water running while drying hands;

f. Dry hands with the clean, disposable paper or single-use cloth towel;

g. If taps do not shut off automatically, turn taps off with a disposable paper or single-use cloth towel;

h. Throw the disposable paper towel into a lined trash container; or place single-use cloth towels in the laundry hamper; or hang individually labeled cloth towels to dry. Use hand lotion to prevent chapping of hands, if desired.

The use of alcohol-based hand sanitizers is an alternative to traditional handwashing with soap and water by children over twenty-four months of age and adults on hands that are not visibly soiled. A single pump of an alcohol-based sanitizer should be dispensed. Hands should be rubbed together, distributing sanitizer to all hand and finger surfaces, and hands should be permitted to air dry.

Situations/times that children and staff should wash their hands should be posted in all handwashing areas.

Use of antimicrobial soap is not recommended in child care settings. There are no data to support use of antibacterial soaps over other liquid soaps.

Children and staff who need to open a door to leave a bathroom or diaper-changing area should open the door with a disposable towel to avoid possibly re-contaminating clean hands. If a child cannot open the door or turn off the faucet, they should be assisted by an adult.

RATIONALE:

Running water over the hands removes visible soil. Wetting the hands before applying soap helps to create a lather that can loosen soil. The soap lather loosens soil and brings it into solution on the surface of the skin. Rinsing the lather off into a sink removes the soil from the hands that the soap brought into solution. Warm water, between 60°F and 120°F, is more comfortable than cold water; using warm water also promotes adequate rinsing during handwashing (1).

Acceptable forms of soap include liquid and powder.

COMMENTS:

Premoistened cleansing towelettes do not effectively clean hands and should not be used as a substitute for washing hands with soap and running water. When running water is unavailable or impractical, the use of alcohol-based hand sanitizer (Standard 3.2.2.5) is a suitable alternative.

Outbreaks of disease have been linked to shared wash water and wash basins (4). Water basins should not be used as an alternative to running water. Camp sinks and portable commercial sinks with foot or hand pumps dispense water as for a plumbed sink and are satisfactory if filled with fresh water daily. The staff should clean and disinfect the water reservoir container and water catch basin daily.

Single-use towels should be used unless an automatic electric hand-dryer is available.

The use of cloth roller towels is not recommended for the following reasons:

a. Children often use cloth roll dispensers improperly, resulting in more than one child using the same section of towel; and

b. Incidents of unintentional strangulation have been reported (U.S. Consumer Product Safety Commission Data Office, pers. comm.).

REFERENCES:

1. Donowitz, L. G., ed. 1996. *Infection Control in the Child Care Center and Preschool,* 2nd ed. Baltimore, MD: Williams and Wilkins.

2. Centers for Disease Control and Prevention. 2011. Handwashing: Clean hands save lives. http://www.cdc.gov/handwashing/.

3. McNeil, S. A., C. L. Foster, S. A. Hedderwick, and C. A. Kauffman. 2001. "Effect of hand cleansing with antimicrobial soap or alcohol-based gel on microbial colonization of artificial fingernails worn by health care workers." *Clin Infect Dis* 32:367–72.

4. Ogunsola, F. T., and Y. O. Adesiji. 2008. "Comparison of four methods of hand washing in situations of inadequate water supply." *West Afr J Med* 27:24–28.

Immunization Schedule

Recommended immunization schedule for persons aged 0 through 6 years—United States, 2012

Vaccine ▼ Age▶	Birth	1 month	2 months	4 months	6 months	9 months	12 months	15 months	18 months	19–23 months	2–3 years	4–6 years
Hepatitis B[1]	HepB	HepB			HepB							
Rotavirus[2]			RV	RV	RV[2]							
Diphtheria, tetanus, pertussis[3]			DTaP	DTaP	DTaP		see footnote[3]	DTaP				DTaP
Haemophilus influenzae type b[4]			Hib	Hib	Hib[4]		Hib					
Pneumococcal[5]			PCV	PCV	PCV		PCV					PPSV
Inactivated poliovirus[6]			IPV	IPV	IPV							IPV
Influenza[7]					Influenza (Yearly)							
Measles, mumps, rubella[8]							MMR		see footnote[8]			MMR
Varicella[9]							Varicella		see footnote[9]			Varicella
Hepatitis A[10]							Dose 1[10]				HepA Series	
Meningococcal[11]							MCV4—see footnote[11]					

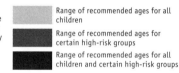

Range of recommended ages for all children

Range of recommended ages for certain high-risk groups

Range of recommended ages for all children and certain high-risk groups

This schedule includes recommendations in effect as of December 23, 2011. Any dose not administered at the recommended age should be administered at a subsequent visit, when indicated and feasible. The use of a combination vaccine generally is preferred over separate injections of its equivalent component vaccines. Vaccination providers should consult the relevant Advisory Committee on Immunization Practices (ACIP) statement for detailed recommendations, available online at http://www.cdc.gov/vaccines/pubs/acip-list.htm. Clinically significant adverse events that follow vaccination should be reported to the Vaccine Adverse Event Reporting System (VAERS) online (http://www.vaers.hhs.gov) or by telephone (800-822-7967).

1. Hepatitis B (HepB) vaccine. (Minimum age: birth)
At birth:
- Administer monovalent HepB vaccine to all newborns before hospital discharge.
- For infants born to hepatitis B surface antigen (HBsAg)-positive mothers, administer HepB vaccine and 0.5 mL of hepatitis B immune globulin (HBIG) within 12 hours of birth. These infants should be tested for HBsAg and anti-body to HBsAg (anti-HBs) 1 to 2 months after completion of at least 3 doses of the HepB series, at age 9 through 18 months (generally at the next well-child visit).
- If mother's HBsAg status is unknown, within 12 hours of birth administer HepB vaccine for infants weighting >2,000 grams, and HepB vaccine plus HBIG for infants weighting <2,000 grams. Determine mother's HBsAg status as soon as possible and, if she is HBsAg-positive, administer HBIG for infants weighing >2,000 grams (no later than age 1 week).

Doses after the birth dose:
- The second dose should be administered at age 1 to 2 months. Monovalent HepB vaccine should be used for doses administered before age 6 weeks.

- Administration of a total of 4 doses of HepB vaccine is permissible when a combination vaccine containing HepB is administered after the birth dose.
- Infants who did not receive a birth dose should receive 3 doses of a HepB-containing vaccine starting as soon as feasible.
- The minimum interval between dose 1 and dose 2 in 4 weeks, and between dose 2 and 3 is 8 weeks. The final (third or fourth) dose in the HepB vaccine series should be administered no earlier than age 24 weeks and at least 16 weeks after the first dose.

2. Rotavirus (RV) vaccines. (Minimum age: 6 weeks for both RV-1 [Rotarix] and RV-5 [Rota Teq])
- The maximum age for the first dose in the series is 14 weeks, 6 days; and 8 months, 0 days for the final dose in the series. Vaccination should not be initiated for infants aged 15 weeks, 0 days or older.
- If RV-1 (Rotarix) is administered at ages 2 and 4 months, a dose at 6 months is not indicated.

3. Diphtheria and tetanus toxoids and acellular pertussis (DTaP) vaccine. (Minimum age: 6 weeks)

- The fourth dose may be administered as early as age 12 months, provided at least 6 months have elapsed since the third dose.

4. Haemophilus influenzae type b (Hib) conjugate vaccine. (Minimum age: 6 weeks)

- If PRP-OMP (PedvaxHIB or Comvax [HepB-Hib]) is administered at ages 2 and 4 months, a dose at age 6 months is not indicated.
- Hiberix should only be used for the booster (final) dose in children aged 12 months through 4 years.

5. Pneumococcal vaccines. (Minimum age: 6 weeks for pneumococcal conjugate vaccine [PCV]; 2 years for pneumococcal polysaccharide vaccine [PPSV])

- Administer 1 dose of PCV to all healthy children aged 24 through 59 months who are not completely vaccinated for their age.
- For children who have received an age-appropriate series of 7-valent PCV (PCV7), a single supplemental dose of 13-valent PCV (PCV13) is recommended for:
  — All children aged 14 through 59 months
  — Children aged 60 through 71 months with underlying medical conditions.
- Administer PPSV at least 8 weeks after last dose of PCV to children aged 2 years or older with certain underlying medical conditions, including a cochlear implant. See MMWR 2010:59(No. RR-11), available at http://www.cdc.gov/mmwr/pdf/rr/rr5911.pdf.

6. Inactivated poliovirus vaccine (IPV). (Minimum age: 6 weeks)

- If 4 or more doses are administered before age 4 years, an additional dose should be administered at age 4 through 6 years.
- The final dose in the series should be administered on or after the fourth birthday and at least 6 months after the previous dose.

7. Influenza vaccines. (Minimum age: 6 months for trivalent inactivated influenza vaccine [TIV]; 2 years for live, attenuated influenza vaccine [LAIV])

- For most healthy children aged 2 years and older, either LAIV or TIV may be used. However, LAIV should not be administered to some children, including 1) children with asthma, 2) children 2 through 4 years who had wheezing in the past 12 months, or 3) children who have any other underlying medical conditions that predispose them to influenza complications. For all other contraindications to use of LAIV, see MMWR 2010;59(No. RR-8), available at http://www.cdc.gov/mmwr/pdf/rr/rr5908.pdf.
- For children aged 6 months through 8 years:
  — For the 2011-12 season, administer 2 doses (separated by at least 4 weeks) to those who did not receive at least 1 dose of the 101-11 vaccine. Those who received at least 1 dose of the 2010-11 vaccine require 1 dose for the 2011-12 season.
  — For the 2012-13 season, follow dosing guidelines in the 2012 ACIP influenza vaccine recommendations.

8. Measles, mumps, and rubella (MMR) vaccine. (Minimum age: 12 months)

- The second dose may be administered before age 4 years, provided at least 4 weeks have elapsed since the first dose.
- Administer MMR vaccine to infants aged 6 through 11 months who are traveling internationally. These children should be revaccinated with 2 doses of MMR vaccine, the first at ages 12 through 15 months and at least 4 weeks after the previous dose, and the second at ages 4 through 6 years.

9. Varicella (VAR) vaccine. (Minimum age: 12 months)

- The second dose may be administered before age 4 years, provided at least 3 months have elapsed since the first dose.
- For children aged 12 months through 12 years, the recommended minimum interval between doses is 3 months. However, if the second dose was administered at least 4 weeks after the first does, it can be accepted as valid.

10. Hepatitis A (HepA) vaccine. (Minimum age: 12 months)

- Administer the second (final) dose 6 to 18 months after the first.
- Unvaccinated children 24 months and older at high risk should be vaccinated. See MMWR 2006;55(No. RR-7), available at http://www.cdc.gov/mmwr/pdf/rr/rr5507.pdf.
- A 2-dose HepA vaccine series is recommended for anyone aged 24 months and older, previously unvaccinated, for whom immunity against hepatitis A virus infection is desired.

11. Meningococcal conjugate vaccines, quadrivalent (MCV4). (Minimum age: 9 months for Menactra [MCV4-D], 2 years for Menveo [MCV4-CRM])

- For children aged 9 through 23 months 1) with persistent complement component deficiency; 2) who are residents of or travelers to countries with hyperendemic or epidemic disease; or 3) who are present during outbreaks caused by vaccine serogroup, administer 2 primary doses of MCV4-D, ideally at ages 9 months and 12 months or at least 8 weeks apart.
- For children aged 24 months and older with 1) persistent complement component deficiency who have not been previously vaccinated; or 2) anatomic/functional asplenia, administer 2 primary doses of either MCV4 at least 8 weeks apart.
- For children with anatomic//functional asplenia, if MCV4-D (Menactra) is used, administer at a minimum age of 2 years and at least 4 weeks after completion of all PCV doses.
- See MMWR 2011;60:72-6, available at http://www.cdc.gov/mmwr/pdf/wk/mm6003.pdf, and Vaccines for Children Program resolution No. 6/11-1, available at http://www.cdc.gov/vaccines/programs/vfc/downloads/resolutions/06-11mening-mcv.pdf, and MMWR 2011;60:1391-2, available at http://www.cdc.gov/mmwr/pdf/wk/mm6040.pdf, for further guidance, including revaccination guidelines.

This schedule is approved by the Advisory Committee on Immunization Practices (http://www.cdc.gove/vaccines/recs/acip), the American Academy of Pediatrics (http:// www.aap.org), and the American Academy of Family Physicians (http://www.aafp.org). Department of Health and Human Services • Centers for Disease Control and Prevention

Moderate and Vigorous Activities for Young Children

	Infants	Toddlers	Preschoolers and school-age
Examples of Moderate Activity	Stretches, tummy time	Practice hopping or jumping, climbing on play equipment, playing stop-and-go games like Going on a Bear Hunt, balance beam, parachute games	Child yoga, monkey bars, hopscotch, riding tricycles, playing stop-and-go games like Red Light, Green Light, skipping or galloping, obstacle courses, parachute games
Examples of Vigorous Activity	Crawling or walking practice, dancing	Running, dancing, prolonged games, activities that require constant action, such as running like different animals or action songs	Games that require prolonged action, such as tag or soccer, or activities that persist for prolonged periods, such as jumping jacks, hula hoop, dancing, running

Adapted from the *2008 Physical Activity Guidelines for Americans.* U.S. Department of Health and Human Services. www.health.gov /paguidelines/guidelines/chapter3.aspx.

MyPlate

Make half your plate fruits and vegetables

Fruits—Any fruit or 100% fruit juice counts as part of the Fruit Group. Fruits may be fresh, canned, frozen, or dried, and may be whole, cut up, or pureed.

Vegetables—Any vegetable or 100% vegetable juice counts as a member of the Vegetable Group. Vegetables may be raw or cooked; fresh, frozen, canned, or dried/dehydrated; and may be whole, cut up, or mashed. Vegetables are divided further into five subgroups. It's important to know which vegetables are most nutritious and strive for variety.

Grains—Any food made from wheat, rice, oats, cornmeal, barley, or another cereal grain

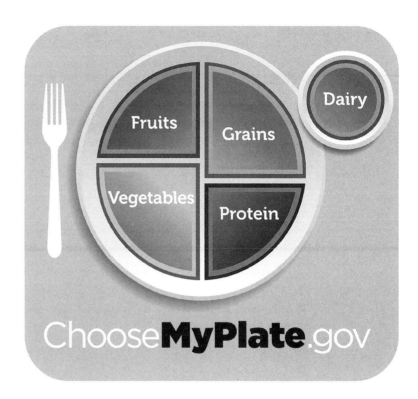

is a grain product. Bread, pasta, oatmeal breakfast cereals, tortillas, and grits are examples of grain products. Grains are divided into two subgroups: whole grains and refined grains. Whole grains contain the entire grain kernel—the bran, germ, and endosperm. Examples of whole grains are: whole wheat flour, oatmeal, brown rice, bulgur. Refined grains have been milled, a process that removes the bran and germ. This is done to give grains a finer texture and improve their shelf life, but it also removes fiber, iron, and many B vitamins. Examples of refined grains are white flour, white bread, and white rice.

Protein—All foods made from meat, poultry, seafood, beans and peas, eggs, processed soy products, nuts, and seeds are considered part of the Protein Foods Group. For more information on beans and peas, see Beans and Peas Are Unique Foods (http://www.choosemyplate.gov/food -groups/vegetables-beans-peas.html).

Select a variety of protein foods to improve nutrient intake and healthy benefits, including at least 8 ounces of cooked seafood per week. Young children need less, depending on their age and calorie needs. The advice to consume seafood doesn not apply to vegetarians. Vegetarian options in the Protein Foods Group include beans and peas, processed soy products, and nuts and seeds. Meat and poultry choices should be lean or low-fat.

Dairy—All fluid milk products and many foods made from milk are considered part of this food group. Most Dairy Group choices should be fat-free or low-fat. Foods made from milk that retain their calcium content are part of the group. Foods made from milk that have little to no calcium, such as cream cheese, cream, and butter, are not. Calcium-fortified soymilk (soy beverage) is also part of the Dairy Group.

NAEYC Accreditation Standards Teacher-Child Ratios within Group Sizes

Age Category	Group Size									
	6	8	10	12	14	16	18	**20**	**22**	**24**
Infant										
Birth to 15 months[b]	1:3	1:4								
Toddler/Two (12–36 months)[b]										
12 to 18 months	1:3	1:4	1:4[c]	1:4						
21 to 36 months		1:4	1:5	1:6						
Preschool[b]										
2½-year-olds to 3-year-olds (30–48 months)				1:6	1:7	1:8	1:9			
4-year-olds						1:8	1:9	1:10		
5-year-olds						1:8	1:9	1:10		
Kindergarten[d]								1:10	1:11	1:12

Notes: In a mixed-age preschool group of 2½-year-olds to 5-year-olds, no more than four children between the ages of 30 months and 36 months may be enrolled. The ratios within group size for the predominant age category apply. If infants or toddlers are in a mixed-age group, then the ratio for the youngest child applies.

Ratios are to be lowered when one or more children in the group need additional adult assistance to fully participate in the program: (1) because of ability, language fluency, developmental age or stage, or other factors, or (2) to meet other requirements of NAEYC Accreditation.

Group sizes as stated are ceilings, regardless of the number of staff.

Ratios and group sizes are always assessed during site visits for NAEYC Accreditation in criterion 10.B.12, which is not a required criterion.

However, experience suggests that programs that exceed the recommended number of children for each teaching staff member and total group sizes will find it more difficult to meet each standard and achieve NAEYC Accreditation. The more these numbers are exceeded, the more difficult it will be to meet each standard.

a. Includes teachers, assistant teachers–teacher aides; some exceptions may apply (see *Determining Teacher-Child Ratios within Group Size*).

b. These age ranges purposefully overlap. If a group includes children whose ages range beyond the overlapping portion of two age categories, then the group is a mixed-age group. For mixed-age groups, universal criteria and criteria relevant to the age categories for that group apply.

c. Group sizes of 10 for this age category would require an additional adult.

d. Kindergarten refers to children enrolled in a public or private kindergarten program.

Nutritional Plan for Infants

If licensing requires or the program has developed a form that meets these same goals, that form can be used. To be updated each month during the first year.

Child's Name: _____   **Date:** _____

What is your child's typical daily feeding schedule?

Time	Type and amount of fluids or food consumed

1. Would you prefer we follow this schedule or feed your child on demand? (Circle one.)

   Schedule   On Demand   Other (describe below)

2. If you choose schedule, please note that it is our policy to feed infants when they show signs of hunger and/or distress; the schedule may therefore fluctuate.

3. If you are breast-feeding your infant or providing expressed breast milk, please indicate how we can best support you:

4. If you are exclusively breast-feeding your child, please outline your daily schedule:

5. If you are exclusively breast-feeding your child, please provide back-up milk in case you are delayed for a scheduled feeding.

6. If your child is eating baby food or table food, please indicate any preferences you have. If you haven't yet introduced solids but plan to do so, please let us know how we can support your efforts.

7. How else can we help you meet your nutritional goals for your infant?

8. Juice and water policy: Please note that our program can only provide milk or formula in bottles. No juice will be given in bottles. Water will be offered in sippy cups for older infants if needed.

9. Food policies: Please note that we do not serve dessert items to infants in baby food or table food. Additionally, our program will not feed solids to infants before four months without a physician's note.

Parent Signature: _____ Date:_____

Proper Handling and Storage of Human Milk

By following safe preparation and storage techniques, nursing mothers and caretakers of breast-fed infants and children can maintain the high quality of expressed breast milk and the health of the baby.

Safely Preparing and Storing Expressed Breast Milk

- Be sure to wash your hands before expressing or handling breast milk.

- When collecting milk, be sure to store it in clean containers, such as screw cap bottles, hard plastic cups with tight caps, or heavy-duty bags that fit directly into nursery bottles. Avoid using ordinary plastic storage bags or formula bottle bags, as these could easily leak or spill.

- If delivering breast milk to a child care provider, clearly label the container with the child's name and date.

- Clearly label the milk with the date it was expressed to facilitate using the oldest milk first.

- Do not add fresh milk to already frozen milk within a storage container. It is best not to mix the two.

- Do not save milk from a used bottle for use at another feeding.

Safely Thawing Breast Milk

- As time permits, thaw frozen breast milk by transferring it to the refrigerator for thawing or by swirling it in a bowl of warm water.

- Avoid using a microwave oven to thaw or heat bottles of breast milk.

  - Microwave ovens do not heat liquids evenly. Uneven heating could easily scald a baby or damage the milk.

  - Bottles may explode if left in the microwave too long.

  - Excess heat can destroy the nutrient quality of the expressed milk.

- Do not refreeze breast milk once it has been thawed.

Storage Duration of Fresh Human Milk for Use with Healthy Full-Term Infants

Location	Temperature	Duration	Comments
Countertop, table	Room temperature (up to 77°F or 25°C)	6–8 hours	Containers should be covered and kept as cool as possible; covering the container with a cool towel may keep the milk cooler.
Insulated cooler bag	5–39°F or -15–4°C	24 hours	Keep ice packs in contact with milk containers at all times, limit opening cooler bag.
Refrigerator	39°F or 4°C	5 days	Store milk in the back of the main body of the refrigerator.
Freezer			
Freezer compartment of a refrigerator	5°F or -15°C	2 weeks	Store milk toward the back of the freezer, where temperature is most constant. Milk stored for longer durations in the ranges listed is safe, but some of the lipids in the milk undergo degradation resulting in lower quality.
Freezer compartment of refrigerator with separate doors	0°F or -18°C	3–6 months	
Chest or upright deep freezer	-4°F or -20°C	6–12 months	
Reference: Academy of Breastfeeding Medicine. (2004) Clinical Protocol Number #8: Human Milk Storage Information for Home Use for Healthy Full-Term Infants. Princeton Junction, New Jersey: Academy of Breastfeeding Medicine.			

Centers for Disease Control and Prevention www.cdc.gov/breastfeeding/recommendations/handling_breastmilk.htm

Routine Schedule for Cleaning, Sanitizing, and Disinfecting

Areas	Before Each Use	After Each Use	Daily (At the End of the Day)	Weekly	Monthly	Comments
Food Areas						
• Food preparation surfaces	Clean, Sanitize	Clean, Sanitize				Use a sanitizer safe for food contact
• Eating utensils & dishes		Clean, Sanitize				If washing the dishes and utensils by hand, use a sanitizer safe for food contact as the final step in the process; Use of an automated dishwasher will sanitize
• Tables & highchair trays	Clean, Sanitize	Clean, Sanitize				
• Countertops		Clean	Clean, Sanitize			Use a sanitizer safe for food contact
• Food preparation appliances		Clean	Clean, Sanitize			
• Mixed use tables	Clean, Sanitize					Before serving food
• Refrigerator					Clean	
Child Care Areas						
• Plastic mouthed toys		Clean	Clean, Sanitize			
• Pacifiers		Clean	Clean, Sanitize			Reserve for use by only one child; Use dishwasher or boil for one minute
• Hats			Clean			Clean after each use if head lice are present
• Door & cabinet handles			Clean, Disinfect			

• Floors			Clean		Sweep or vacuum, then damp mop, (consider micro fiber damp mop to pick up most particles)
• Machine washable cloth toys				Clean	Launder
• Dress-up clothes				Clean	Launder
• Play activity centers				Clean	
• Drinking Fountains			Clean, Disinfect		
• Computer keyboards		Clean, Sanitize			Use sanitizing wipes, do not use spray
• Phone receivers			Clean		
Toilet & Diapering Areas					
• Changing tables		Clean, Disinfect			Clean with detergent, rinse, disinfect
• Potty chairs		Clean, Disinfect			
• Handwashing sinks & faucets			Clean, Disinfect		
• Countertops			Clean, Disinfect		
• Toilets			Clean, Disinfect		
• Diaper pails			Clean, Disinfect		
• Floors			Clean, Disinfect		Damp mop with a floor cleaner/ disinfectant
Sleeping Areas					
• Bed sheets & pillowcases				Clean	Clean before use by another child
• Cribs, cots, & mats				Clean	Clean before use by another child
• Blankets					Clean

Additional Resources

American Academy of Pediatrics Childhood Immunization Support Program

http://www2.aap.org/immunization/about/programfacts.html

This website, sponsored by the American Academy of Pediatrics, provides helpful information for professionals and families about childhood immunizations. It contains a printable version of the childhood immunization schedule as well as information to help families understand the importance of childhood immunizations.

Academy of Nutrition and Dietetics

www.eatright.org/Public

This website is a collection of information on all nutrition topics developed by nutrition experts. It contains a plethora of information, including sections on childhood obesity, nutrition for life, and food safety.

Academy of Nutrition and Dietetics: Savvy Food Shopping

www.eatright.org/Public/content.aspx?id=5552

This website offers the following articles: "Save Time and Money at the Grocery Store," "Become a Savvy Farmer's Market Shopper," "Lighten Your Carbon Food Print," and "Shopping with Food Safety."

Action for Healthy Kids

www.actionforhealthykids.org

This nonprofit organization provides tools and resources for schools, families, and communities to promote healthy kids.

***Active for Life: Developmentally Appropriate Movement Programs for Young Children,* by Stephen W. Sanders**

This book addresses the need for early childhood educators to ensure children's learning of physical skills and movement concepts. If young children learn physical activity concepts early on, they will build a foundation of skills for years to come. It also provides information on what high-quality movement programs should include.

American Academy of Pediatrics—Childhood Immunization Support Program

www2.aap.org/immunization/about/programfacts.html

This website, sponsored by the American Academy of Pediatrics, provides helpful information about immunizations. Providers and parents will find the "Immunization Schedule" and "Vaccine Safety" sections particularly helpful. Providers can find research-based information to share with parents who may be reluctant about childhood immunizations and their safety.

American Academy of Pediatrics—Emotional Wellness

www.healthychildren.org/English/healthy-living/emotional-wellness/Pages/default.aspx

This website has articles and resources on a plethora of topics related to childhood emotions and emotional health.

American Academy of Pediatrics—Policy Statement

http://pediatrics.aappublications.org/content/early/2011/10/12/peds.2011-1753

This 2011 policy statement addresses media use for children under age two. It lists key evidence for their recommendations for television viewing for the youngest children. There are recommendations for parents as well as child care professionals.

Best Practice for Healthy Eating: A Guide to Helping Children Grow up Healthy

www.nemours.org/content/dam/nemours/www/filebox/service/preventive/nhps/heguide.pdf

This downloadable brochure has information and visuals that are easy to understand and use. The brochure covers portion sizes for children, food item ideas, first meals, working with picky eaters, and more.

Caring for Our Children: National Health and Safety Performance Standards: Guidelines for Early Care and Education Programs, 3rd edition, by AAP, APHA, and NRC

Available online at http://nrckids.org

The full text of the national standards can be found online at the National Resource Center for Health and Safety in Child Care and Early Education. The standards and accompanying text describe the best practices for promoting health and safety in early care and education programs as well as the research supporting each standard. Standards on the website are routinely updated as new research is conducted.

Center on the Social and Emotional Foundations for Early Learning (CSEFEL)

http://csefel.vanderbilt.edu

CSEFEL is a national resource center funded by the Office of Head Start and Child Care Bureau for disseminating research- and evidence-based practices to early childhood programs across the country focused on promoting the social and emotional development and school readiness of young children from birth to age five.

Child Care Exchange

www.childcareexchange.com

This website contains articles from the popular magazine *Exchange* and other resources for program leaders. Using the website, program leaders can register for *ExchangeEveryDay*, a free daily e-mail message on a wide range of leadership topics in early care and education.

Child Welfare Information Gateway

www.childwelfare.gov

This website, sponsored by the U.S. Department of Health and Human Services, provides information about child abuse and neglect including tools for recognizing and reporting child abuse, supporting families, and providing family education. The site has up-to-date statistics on child abuse incidence and a number of helpful resources that can be downloaded or ordered.

Choosy Kids

www.choosykids.com/CK2

This website is a curriculum tool for home and child care programs that focuses on helping kids be healthier and learn healthy habits. There are products for sale, training opportunities, and resources for parents and teachers.

Color Me Healthy

www.colormehealthy.com

Color Me Healthy is a nutrition curriculum that can be purchased from the North Carolina State University and A&T State University extension offices. The program is aimed at four- and five-year-olds. Through fun, interactive learning opportunities, children learn that physical activity and eating healthy food are fun.

CPSC—Crib Information Center

www.cpsc.gov/info/cribs/index.html

This website, developed and maintained by the U.S. Consumer Product Safety Commission, provides detailed information about safe cribs. Programs can sign up for crib recall notifications and search information about new crib standards. A number of downloadable posters and other resources are also available on the website, including an excellent "checklist for safe sleep" poster.

CPSC—Product Recalls

www.cpsc.gov/cpscpub/prerel/prerel.html

The U.S. Consumer Product Safety Commission's website gathers important information about a wide range of product recalls. Providers can search for recalled items or review recent announcements of product recalls. Recall notices are grouped in categories, including "children's products" and "toys." Providers can also sign up to receive electronic notifications of recalled products.

The Devereux Early Childhood Initiative
http://www.devereux.org/site/PageServer?pagename=deci_index

This organization has a continuum of strengths-based assessments and planning systems designed to promote resilience in young children. They also have tools to assess and promote resilience in caregivers.

Early Childhood Learning & Knowledge Center
http://eclkc.ohs.acf.hhs.gov/hslc/tta-system/health/ep

This website, sponsored by the U.S. Department of Health and Human Services for use by Head Start programs, contains information that is helpful to all early childhood programs. The "Health" landing page includes information on a broad range of potential emergencies (tornado, flood, earthquake, etc.). Programs can search by topic for user-friendly information created specifically for early childhood programs.

Einstein Never Used Flashcards, by Kathy Hirsh-Pasek, PhD, Roberta Michnick Golinkoff, and Diane Eyer
This book includes multiple stories and examples describing why rote memorization, worksheets, and other drill practice activities are useless and even harmful to young children. This book is useful to teachers and parents alike.

Enthusiastic and Engaged Learners: Approaches to Learning in the Early Childhood Classroom, by Marilou Hyson
Approaches to learning, or learning dispositions, are the least understood learning domain and thus typically receive the least attention. This book provides an in-depth look at approaches to learning and provides practical ideas for the classroom.

FEMA—Earthquake Preparedness: What Every Child Care Provider Needs to Know
www.fema.gov/library/viewRecord.do?id=1520

This booklet, developed by the U.S. Department of Homeland Security, Federal Emergency Management Agency (FEMA), provides checklists and information for programs about what to do before, during, and after an earthquake. Helpful resources include instruction on "Drop, Cover, and Hold," and a checklist for an earthquake emergency kit.

Follow Me Too: A Handbook of Movement Activities for Three- to Five-Year-Olds, by Marianne Torbert and Lynne Schneider
Movement activities encourage cooperative learning and teamwork. This book includes research and the theory behind using movement games, field-tested games, adaptations for individual abilities and needs, a chart of skills involved in each game, ideas for parent involvement, and information on how to make inexpensive equipment.

Fred Rogers Center for Early Learning and Children's Media

www.fredrogerscenter.org

This organization is devoted to using the potential of media to enhance children's experiences without harming their development. The website provides many articles and research papers.

The Fred Rogers Company

www.fci.org/new-site/professional.html

This organization focuses on providing the field with resources and tools to best understand and support children's social and emotional development and wellness.

Go Green Rating Scale for Early Childhood Settings and *Go Green Rating Scale for Early Childhood Settings Handbook: Improving Your Score,* by Phil Boise

These two books, available from Redleaf Press (www.redleafpress.org), offer in-depth resources and a useful rating scale that addresses environmental health and safety. Programs can rate their facility and practices in nine areas: administration, green living and stewardship, cleaners and disinfectants, body-care and hygiene products, air-quality management, exposure to lead, exposure to chemicals found in plastics, pesticides, and other contaminants. The handbook in particular offers a wealth of research-based information and resources for program improvement.

Growing, Growing Strong: A Whole Health Curriculum for Young Children, by Connie Jo Smith, Charlotte M. Hendricks, and Becky S. Bennett

This health curriculum is full of practical ideas and information. It includes lesson plans and interactive activities. With topics such as body parts, the five senses, eating healthy foods, emotions, and friendships, the book aims at teaching young children about their bodies and how to care for them.

Head Start Emergency Preparedness Manual

http://eclkc.ohs.acf.hhs.gov/hslc/tta-system/health/ep/Head_Start_Emergency_Preparedness_Manual.pdf

All programs benefit from emergency preparedness planning. Head Start has created a detailed resource to assist its programs in preparing for a wide range of emergencies. The manual is available online and can help programs of all types in their planning. The manual includes helpful worksheets, checklists, and examples.

Healthy Child Care—International Child Resource Institute

www.globalhealthychildcare.dreamhosters.com

This resource-rich website provides information on how to create healthy and safe environments for young children. It has a wide range of health- and safety-related materials, including a program for self-assessment, self-guided training modules, and downloadable posters for hand washing, diapering, and cleaning and sanitizing the environment. Materials are available in several languages.

I Am Moving, I Am Learning

http://eclkc.ohs.acf.hhs.gov/hslc/tta-system/health/Health/Nutrition/Nutrition Program Staff/IamMovingIam.htm

I Am Moving, I Am Learning is a nutrition and physical activity curriculum for Head Start and Early Start grantees. It addresses childhood obesity in Head Start children. The curriculum aims to increase physical activity, improve the quality of activities planned and facilitated by adults, and encourage healthy food choices.

KidsHealth

http://kidshealth.org

This website has excellent resources for parents, educators, and kids on all topics related to health and nutrition. It has a parents', kids', and teens' site. It is full of brief, easy-to-read articles on all topics related to children's health, including nutrition and physical activity.

KidsHealth—Emotions

http://kidshealth.org/parent/emotions/index.html

This online collection of resources from Nemours includes engaging and short resources for parents and educators about typical child emotions and behaviors (also cited in the nutrition and physical fitness sections).

Learning Zone Xpress—Nutrition Education Products

www.learningzonexpress.com

This website provides many child care–friendly resources, posters, lesson plans, stickers, DVDs, and activity ideas related to nutrition and fitness. It has products on nutrition, child development, culinary topics, fashion and design, go green activities, health activities, and life skills. Spanish products are also available.

Let's Move! Child Care

http://healthykidshealthyfuture.org/welcome.html

This website includes First Lady Michelle Obama's initiative to reverse the trends of childhood obesity in a generation. There is information about getting started with healthy eating and physical activities. Tools and links to great resources for child care providers as well as families are also included.

Little Kids, Big Worries: Stress-Busting Tips for Early Childhood Classrooms, by Alice Sterling Honig

Included in this book are an explanation of how stressful events affect children, what adults can do to protect them from the affects of stress, and advice to help them through stressful situations.

The "Loving Support" Program—WIC

www.nal.usda.gov/wicworks/Learning_Center/support_bond.html

This program promotes and supports breast-feeding. There are many PDFs available to download, including a project summary, posters, and brochures that discuss myths and barriers associated with breast-feeding.

Magic Capes, Amazing Powers: Transforming Superhero Play in the Classroom, by Eric Hoffman

Anyone who has worked with young children has encountered a "superhero" or two before. This resource provides information and strategies about superhero play. It discusses why children are attracted to superhero play, why parents and teachers are concerned, and what strategies teachers can use to guide superhero play in a way that allows children to play and addresses adult concerns.

Managing Chronic Health Needs in Child Care and Schools: A Quick Reference Guide, edited by Elaine A. Donoghue, MD, and Colleen A. Kraft, MD

This book, developed by the American Academy of Pediatrics, addresses care plans for children with chronic health needs. It also provides thorough information about best practices for medication administration. An A to Z collection of quick reference sheets on health needs, such as allergies, diabetes, autism, and seizures, is helpful for a wide range of programs. The book also includes sample forms and documents, such as emergency information forms for children with special health needs and asthma treatment plans.

Managing Infectious Diseases in Child Care and Schools: A Quick Reference Guide edited by Susan S. Aronson and Timothy R. Shope

This book, published by the American Academy of Pediatrics, provides a wealth of information in an easy-to-read format. The book addresses ways to prevent, identify, and respond to infectious diseases. The Quick Reference Sheets are a particularly helpful tool in communicating with families and staff members.

McCormick Center for Early Childhood Leadership

http://cecl.nl.edu/index.htm

This website provides a range of excellent information helpful to program leaders. The website contains information about helpful assessment tools, the Early Childhood Work Environment

Survey, the Program Administration Scale (PAS), and the Business Administration Scale (BAS), and links to professional development for program leaders. Program leaders will find the archive of *The Director's Link* newsletters extremely helpful.

McCormick Center for Early Childhood Leadership—Early Childhood Work Environment Survey

http://cecl.nl.edu/evaluation/resources/ecwes_short.pdf

The Early Childhood Work Environment Survey is a measure of the organization climate in a program. The survey is used with employees in a program to understand their perceptions of ten dimensions of work climate. The full version of the survey is available online through the McCormick Center for Early Childhood Leadership, and in the book *A Great Place to Work: Creating a Healthy Organizational Climate* by Paula Jorde Bloom, Ann Hentschel, and Jill Bella. A short version of the survey can be downloaded for free.

Medical Emergencies in Early Childhood Settings: A Quick Reference Guide, by Charlotte Hendricks

This book, published by Redleaf Press, is an excellent supplement to first aid training and contains short, on-the-spot advice for addressing emergencies such as nosebleeds, choking, allergic reactions, and fever. It also gives advice on when to call paramedics, tells how to make a first aid kit, and offers prevention tips for child care environments.

Mind in the Making: The Seven Essential Life Skills Every Child Needs, by Ellen Galinsky

This book is written for both teachers and parents, detailing the seven essential life skills children need to be successful. Galinsky evaluates the findings of multiple research studies and translates the results into easy-to-read language. She provides sample activities that can be done with children to promote these skills.

Moving and Learning

www.movingandlearning.com

This program developed by Rae Pica, a notable early childhood expert, includes physical activity resources, ideas, and information for children from birth through eight years old. The website offers articles, activities, and other resources.

NAEYC—*Keeping Healthy: Families, Teachers, and Children*

This trifold brochure is available for purchase from the National Association for the Education of Young Children (www.naeyc.org). The brochure addresses hand washing, cleaning, immunizations, diapering, and illness prevention. It includes an abbreviated version of a cleaning and sanitizing schedule. Programs will find this brochure useful in staff training and as a resource to share with families.

National Heart, Lung, and Blood Institute: We Can! Resources

www.nhlbi.nih.gov/health/public/heart/obesity/wecan/index.htm

The We Can! resources are a collection of materials that can be shared with families and/or used in a program. The resources are all about how to help children maintain a healthy weight. The information is interesting, and the resources are user-friendly.

National Resource Center for Health and Safety in Child Care and Early Education—Motion Moments

http://nrckids.org/Motion_Moments/index.htm

This website provides free, short, how-to video clips on adding more movement into a program. The children in the videos include infants, toddlers, and preschoolers. There are also additional resources focused on movement for infants, toddlers, and preschoolers.

National Resource Center for Health and Safety in Child Care and Early Education—State Licensing and Regulation Information

http://nrckids.org/STATES/states.htm

This landing page of the National Resource Center for Health and Safety in Child Care and Early Education links programs to up-to-date information about child care regulations in every state. To find regulations for an individual state, click on the state, and you will find the most recent version of regulations pertaining to child care and early education posted as links.

Nurturing Young Children's Dispositions to Learn, by Sara Wilford

This resource connects multiple factors that influence children's learning and development, such as learning styles, brain development, and multiple intelligences, and explains how to nurture skills and dispositions children need most to help them learn and thrive.

The Nutrition and Physical Activity Self-Assessment for Child Care (NAP SACC)

www.center-trt.org/index.cfm?fa=opinterventions.intervention&intervention=napsacc&page=intent

This organization offers resources and training for programs. It offers free online training on nutrition and physical activity topics. The training provides an in-depth, but practical, understanding of these topics.

Office of Head Start Emergency Preparedness Manual

http://eclkc.ohs.acf.hhs.gov/hslc/tta-system/health/ep/Head_Start_Emergency_Preparedness_Manual.pdf

This manual, created by the federal Office of Head Start, is an excellent example for programs developing emergency policies and procedures. The entire manual is available online. The manual addresses preparation for emergencies such as weather-related emergencies, health emergencies, and more.

The Power of Guidance: Teaching Social-Emotional Skills in Early Childhood Classrooms and *A Guidance Approach for the Encouraging Classroom,* by Dan Gartrell

Gartrell is an expert in children's challenging behavior. Considering behavior as a form of communication and behavior guidance as a way to teach children the skills they need to make better decisions about behavior, Gartrell provides practical and applicable tips and strategies to effectively support children.

The Power of Play: Learning What Comes Naturally, by David Elkind

This book helps teachers and parents understand the power of play and identifies exactly how much children are learning when they do engage in play. Through research analysis and examples, Elkind shows how play promotes healthy mental and social development and how it helps children get ready for academic learning.

Program Administration Scale: Measuring Early Childhood Leadership and Management, by Teri N. Talan and Paula Jorde Bloom

This book contains a research-based rating scale for use in understanding ten dimensions of program administration: human resources development, personnel cost and allocation, center operations, child assessment, fiscal management, program planning and evaluation, family partnerships, marketing and public relations, technology, and staff qualifications. Providers can use this tool to understand and improve administrative practices in a center or program.

Prove It! Achieving Quality Recognition for Your Early Childhood Program, by Rachel Robertson and Miriam Dressler

This book, published by Redleaf Press, offers providers a guide for improving program quality. The book includes helpful information on assessing, setting goals, and improving quality in areas including health and safety and learning environments.

Public Playground Safety Handbook
www.cpsc.gov/cpscpub/pubs/325.pdf

This publication, developed by the U.S. Consumer Products Safety Commission, is available entirely online. The manual lists the ASTM playground safety standards and provides general considerations of developing, designing, and maintaining a playground for young children.

Raising Resilient Children Foundation
http://www.raisingresilientkids.com/index.html

This website provides information to help adults raise, support, and develop stress-hardy children. There is a resiliency quiz, book, and videos, and resources and information about this topic.

Recognizing Common Illnesses in Early Childhood Settings, by Hilary Pert Stecklein, MD

This book, available from Redleaf Press (www.readleafpress.org), is an excellent resource for staff training and a helpful supplement to first aid training. The book addresses common symptoms of childhood illnesses as well as illness prevention topics.

Safe Kids USA—Car Seats, Boosters, and Seat Belt Safety

http://www.safekids.org/safety-basics/safety-resources-by-risk-area
/car-seats-boosters-seat-belts/

This website contains up-to-date information about child restraint requirements as well as helpful tips for choosing and using child safety restraints. There are excellent, free-to-download resources to share with families and to use within programs. For example, the site features a tip sheet on when to turn children from back-facing to front-facing in the car and an excellent video on the importance of child passenger safety.

Sesame Street—Food for Thought: Eating Well on a Budget

www.sesamestreet.org/parents/topicsandactivities/toolkits/food

This bilingual, multimedia program is intended to help support families who have children between the ages of two and eight and are experiencing uncertain or limited access to affordable and nutritious food. All of the links are specific sections of resources recommended for general reference. The links refer to information about eating healthy on a budget.

Sesame Street "Healthy Habits for Life"

www.sesamestreet.org/parents/topicsandactivities/toolkits/healthyhabits

This Sesame Street initiative includes a video, online clips, games, and printable materials featuring some well-loved characters. Research indicates that an endorsement from Elmo can make vegetables appealing to a young child.

Social and Emotional Development: Connecting Science and Practice in Early Childhood Settings, by Dave Riley, Robert R. San Juan, Joan Klinkner, and Ann Ramminger

This easy-to-read overview covers some of the most notable theorists and theories that shape our approach to social and emotional development. It explains not only the research behind many early childhood practices but also the limitations of others.

SPARK

www.sparkpe.org/early-childhood

SPARK seeks to improve the lifelong wellness of children, adolescents, and adults. There are research- and evidence-based programs (for teachers and leaders serving preschool through twelfth grade) for physical education, after school, early childhood, and coordinated school health. Each program includes curricula, on-site teacher training, follow-up support, and equipment.

Strengthening Families

www.strengtheningfamilies.net

Strengthening Families is a structure developed by the Center for the Study of Social Policy (CSSP) to prevent child abuse and neglect. It is a national and state initiative to provide training and support to child care providers that results in the development of protective factors within families.

Technical Assistance Center on Social Emotional Intervention for Young Children (TACSEI)

www.challengingbehavior.org

This website is funded by the U.S. Department of Education. TACSEI translates research on social-emotional outcomes for young children into practical and free products and resources that inform teaching practices. Many resources apply to children at risk for delays or disabilities.

This Emotional Life—Early Moments Matter

www.pbs.org/thisemotionallife/campaign/early-moments-matter

This initiative by PBS provides useful information to parents and families about how to support their child's emotional wellness from the start.

U.S. Department of Agriculture (USDA)—Grow It, Try It, Like It!

www.fns.usda.gov/tn/Resources/growit.html

This resource is an education kit for child care centers that emphasizes growing and trying new fruits and vegetables. The kit includes hands-on activities, planting activities, and nutrition activities. The full booklet is available in PDF.

USDA—*Menu Magic for Children*

www.fns.usda.gov/tn/resources/menumagic.html

This booklet provides information on the Child and Adult Care Food Program (CACFP) Meal Pattern requirements and serving quality meals and snacks, and tips on menu planning and grocery shopping. It is available in PDF. It is a comprehensive resource for child care providers and/or centers or school chefs. Menus, recipes, and substitution ideas are included.

USDA—MyPlate

www.choosemyplate.gov

MyPlate is the updated version of the food pyramid. If you only go to one resource, go to this one. There are myriad tools, resources, and information to use and/or share with families.

USDA—MyPlate: Healthy Eating on a Budget

www.choosemyplate.gov/healthy-eating-on-budget.html

This website provides tips and materials to help you make healthy eating choices on a budget. For example, there is information on eating better on a budget and how to shop for vegetables and fruits on a budget, and a sample weekly menu.

USDA—Nibbles for Health

www.fns.usda.gov/tn/resources/nibbles.html

This website provides nutrition newsletters for parents of young children in child care centers and child care center staff. The sharing sessions (which offer child care center staff guidance on having discussions with parents) and reproducible newsletters are available to download in PDF.

USDA—Recipe Finder

http://recipefinder.nal.usda.gov

This website offers recipes submitted by nutrition and health professionals and organizations. There is a search tool for specific recipes and ingredients.

USDA—Team Nutrition Resource Library

http://teamnutrition.usda.gov/library.html

This website includes a list of all of the resources developed by the USDA related to children's nutrition. There are games, activity books, menu planning, evaluating tools, and much more. The resources are also subdivided by audience.

USDA—*The Two-Bite Club*

www.fns.usda.gov/tn/Resources/2biteclub.html

Parents or caregivers read the book to children and try to inspire them to try new foods from each food group. The back of the book includes additional activities and tips for children. This storybook is available to download in PDF.

The War Play Dilemma: What Every Parent and Teacher Needs to Know, by Diane E. Levin and Nancy Carlsson-Paige

For caregivers looking to understand and identify how to best respond to children's war play, this resource provides an in-depth look at this natural form of "play." The book provides guidance for working with children to promote creative play and for influencing the lessons about violence children are learning. Also, the book includes possible strategies for resolving the war play dilemma.

We Can! GO, SLOW, and WHOA Foods

www.nhlbi.nih.gov/health/public/heart/obesity/wecan/downloads/go-slow-whoa.pdf

A simple but effective one-page chart categorizes foods in three columns: go (eat almost anytime), slow (eat in moderation), and whoa (rarely or never eat). Great for a bulletin board, newsletter, or the fridge.

Women, Infants, and Children (WIC)

www.fns.usda.gov/wic

WIC provides federal grants to states for food, health care referrals, and nutrition education. WIC provides free resources for child nutrition, pregnant mothers, and breast-feeding. WIC is not only for low-income families.

Zero to Three: National Center for Infants, Toddlers, and Families

www.zerotothree.org/child-development/social-emotional-development/social-emotional-development.html

This well-known and well-respected organization focuses on the development of children from ages zero to three. This link leads to their social and emotional development information and resources.

Glossary

allergen: Substance a person is allergic to.

allergy: Abnormal reaction of the immune system to an allergen. The allergy may be one that is eaten, breathed into the lungs, touched, or injected into the body.

antibacterial: Product developed to kill bacteria on surfaces or the body. Antibacterial hand soaps are commonly marketed.

approaches to learning skills: A blend of cognitive and social-emotional skills and abilities that children use to learn and acquire skills and knowledge.

asbestos: Fiber that was used in building materials, such as insulation and floor and ceiling tiles. Also used in some industrial processes, fabrics, decorations, and kitchen equipment.

asthma: Disorder that causes the lungs' airways to swell and narrow, leading to wheezing, shortness of breath, chest tightness, and coughing. Asthma can be triggered by allergens.

attachment: The connection or bond between a child and a caregiver. It describes the sense of safety and security a child feels with an adult. The attachment can be secure or positive, meaning the child can trust and rely on the caregiver; it can be insecure or negative, meaning the caregiver is inconsistent or unavailable, and the child cannot trust or rely on the caregiver.

behavior guidance: A method of preventing or responding to children's behavior that focuses on teaching positive ways to manage, express, and resolve children's thoughts and emotions.

blood-borne pathogens: Bacteria and viruses that can be transmitted only through blood or blood-containing body fluids, such as feces or mucus. Hepatitis is an example of an illness transmitted by blood-borne pathogens.

body mass index (BMI): A weight-to-height ratio, measuring fat in specific areas of the body to assess overall body fat.

cardiopulmonary resuscitation, or CPR: First aid procedure used when a victim is not breathing. May include rescue breathing and chest compressions.

cavities, or dental caries: Holes in teeth resulting from tooth decay. Decay is caused by buildup of plaque, which contains acid-producing bacteria.

child abuse: Defined in federal law as "any recent act or failure to act on the part of a parent or caretaker, which results in death, serious physical or emotional harm, sexual abuse, or exploitation, or; An act or failure to act which presents an imminent risk of serious harm" (U.S. Code 42). States have their own legal definitions of abuse. Most recognize four major types of maltreatment or abuse: physical abuse, neglect, sexual abuse, and emotional abuse.

chronic illnesses or chronic health care needs: Health conditions expected to persist over time and even to last a child's lifetime. Chronic illnesses or chronic health care needs include asthma, diabetes, attention deficit disorder, Down syndrome, allergies, epilepsy, and many, many more.

cleaning: Physically removing dirt and contamination. Cleaning can be accomplished with water and a cloth and does not necessarily require commercial cleaners or other cleaning products.

complex carbohydrates: Complex carbohydrates contain multiple vitamins and minerals. They are harder for the body to break down and don't turn into sugar as readily. Most of a person's daily calorie intake should come from complex carbohydrates. (Lots of information and misinformation about carbohydrates have been published in recent years. For more details on all types of carbohydrates, refer to http://www.nlm.nih.gov/medlineplus/ency/article/002469.htm.)

conversational language: Language used in conversations or back-and-forth exchanges between two or more people.

cross-contamination: Introduction of microorganisms from one surface to another because of faulty hygiene or kitchen practices.

daily recommended value (DRV): The minimum or maximum amount each day of something (vitamin, mineral, sodium, protein, fat, and so on) suggested for a particular group of people by the U.S. Food and Drug Administration. The nationally established values are for children four and over and adults. (Because of varied growth rates, DRVs have not been set for children under four.) Children should have *at least* the DRV of each vitamin and mineral and *no more* than the DRV of sodium, sugars, and fats each day. Sometimes referred to as *DV*, or *daily value*.

DEET: Abbreviation for diethylmetatoluamide, a compound found in many insect repellents.

delayed gratification: The ability to wait for something wanted or desired.

directive language: Used to give instructions or directions. It is typically one-sided and requires little if any response.

discipline: Activities that promote adherence or obedience to rules or expectations.

disinfecting: Killing organisms (germs) such as most bacteria, fungi, molds, and viruses. It is done with commercial products designed to disinfect. True disinfectants must carry product labels that identify the organisms they are designed to kill. Products must be approved by the U.S. Environmental Protection Agency (EPA) as disinfectants.

dwell time: Amount of time a disinfecting product needs to kill target organisms. Disinfecting products may require up to ten minutes of dwell time to be effective. During this time, the surface being disinfected must remain wet. After the dwell time is complete, the surface must be cleaned with water to remove residual disinfectant.

emotional intelligence: Ability to understand one's own (intrapersonal) and others' (interpersonal) emotions, to respond to situations with appropriate emotion, and to regulate emotions. In other words, to perceive, control, and evaluate emotions.

empathy: Capacity to recognize and understand the feelings or experiences of another person.

evacuation: Act of making an emergency exit from the child care space.

evacuation route: Designated path children and adults should take from the child care spaces during an emergency. Each space used by children may have a different evacuation route. The evacuation route should use the most direct exit from the space.

exclusion policy: Conditions under which children must be excluded from group care.

exercise: Physical activity specifically focused on increasing or maintaining fitness.

extrinsic motivation: Motivation or drive inspired by things external to a person, like rewards or prestige.

facility: All of the program's buildings and outdoor areas, including sheds and other storage units.

family-style dining: Meals or snacks eaten as a group while seated at a table. These eating experiences include conversation and healthy eating habits, such as eating more slowly, making choices about foods eaten, and controlling portion sizes. Family-style dining minimizes eating in isolation, which is often associated with overeating.

fever: A body temperature that is elevated above normal. In children, oral temperatures above 101 degrees Fahrenheit, rectal temperatures above 102 degrees Fahrenheit, and axillary (armpit) temperatures above 100 degrees Fahrenheit are considered above normal (AAP 2011, 2).

fire extinguisher: Portable device that emits chemicals as liquids, powders, or foams to put out fires when activated. Fire extinguishers come in many types and require routine maintenance.

fitness: A measurement of a person's physical well-being.

food insecurity: When a person does not have regular access to adequate food or regular meals.

group size: Number of children that can be cared for in a group at one time. A group might require more than one adult caregiver, depending on the ratio of children to adults required for the group. For example, a group size of eight indicates that eight children can be cared for together in a group. Depending on the age of the children, this group size may require two caregivers if the ratio for this group is 1:4.

immunization: Vaccine given to children or adults to help them develop protection against specific infections, such as tuberculosis, measles, mumps, or chicken pox. Immunizations are also referred to as *vaccinations*.

in-service training: Training that accumulates while someone works in a job. In-service training may also be called *continuing education* or *professional development*.

integrated pest management (IPM): Site-specific decision-making process that addresses pest problems with the least impact on human health. Integrated pest management may involve the use of traps, maintenance procedures, and pesticides. It is based on knowledge of pest biology and habitats.

interactive media: Media that require responses, such as computer games or a gaming console, from the viewer.

internal motivation: Motivation or drive inspired by things internal to a person, such as personal goals or values (synonymous with intrinsic motivation).

interpersonal: Of or pertaining to the relations between persons.

intrapersonal: Occurring within the individual mind or self.

lead: Highly toxic metal that used to be used in paint, pottery glazes, and glass. Lead was also present in gasoline until it was phased out in the 1970s. Deposits of lead can be found in groundwater and soil, especially in areas with heavy traffic.

lifeguard: Person specially trained to observe and supervise water activities and to respond to emergency situations in water.

macronutrients: Nutrients that provide calories and energy and are needed in large quantities throughout the day (compared to micronutrients). Macronutrients are carbohydrates, proteins, and fats.

medical home: Place where a child (and family) receives continuous primary medical care. Most children's medical home is a pediatrician with whom they have a long-standing partnership.

micronutrients: Nutrients needed in small amounts through the day. These include vitamins and minerals.

moderate activity: Activity that increases a person's heart rate but causes breathing to become only slightly harder.

monounsaturated fat: A healthy type of fat found in foods and oils, associated with some health benefits such as regulating blood sugar and insulin.

NOAA (National Oceanic and Atmospheric Administration): Federal agency that operates a national network of radio stations transmitting severe-weather warnings, watches, forecasts, and hazard information.

nonprescription medications: See "over-the-counter medications."

nutrient-dense foods: Foods containing a high amount of nutrients compared to their number of calories. For example, carrots are more than twenty times more nutrient dense than potato chips (http://shine.yahoo.com).

nutrients: Substances in food needed to maintain health and support growth. The six essential nutrients needed daily are water, carbohydrates, proteins, fats, vitamins, and minerals.

nutritionally void: Words used to describe foods with minimal or no essential vitamins or nutrients, such as french fries, pastries, and chips.

nutritious: Word used to describe foods and beverages that contain high levels of nutrients.

orientation: Training that occurs immediately after hire. It introduces employees to their positions. Orientation is sometimes also referred to as *on-boarding*.

over-the-counter medications: Drugs sold directly to individuals without direction from a physician. These medications are considered safe when used according to the manufacturer's instructions.

passive media: Media, such as television or movies, that require no participation or interaction from the viewer.

pesticides: Substances used to kill living organisms. Pesticides can be liquids, sprays, powders, or solid substances like baits. They may or may not be registered by the U.S. Environmental Protection Agency (EPA) to kill pests. Pesticide products can be purchased at many retail and commercial outlets. They may be designed for use by a pest control professional or a facility owner or operator.

physical activity: Activity that requires large body movements.

policy: Comprehensive statement of decisions, courses of action, principles, and judgments designed to help programs meet their goals and fulfill their mission.

polyunsaturated fat: A healthy type of fat found in plant-based foods and oils, associated with some health benefits such as lower blood pressure and heart health.

portion: The amount of food a person chooses to eat. For example, a portion of milk is the amount put in a glass to drink.

prescription medication: Drug obtained with specific directions for use, prescribed for a particular individual by a physician.

pre-service training: Training required before working with children.

primary caregiver: Person who cares for a child the most. In an early care and education setting, this refers to the teacher assigned to the child, who is responsible for knowing the child's needs, development, progress, personality, and temperament. The teacher individualizes the child's care and education. This does not preclude other teachers from interacting with the child.

prosocial behavior: Voluntary behavior that contributes to positive social interactions and relationships.

punishment: A hardship someone must endure for something he or she has done. Learning is not the goal of punishment.

ratio: Number of children who can be cared for by one adult. For example, a 4:1 ratio indicates that four children can be cared for by one adult.

receptive/active listening: Method of listening that ensures the speaker's message is heard, understood, and responded to.

resilience: Ability to recover or adapt after a challenge or adversity.

salmonella: Bacterium that causes infections. Salmonella can be transmitted to humans through contact with some animals and their feces and a variety of foods, including eggs, poultry, and contaminated fruits and vegetables.

sanitizing: Reduction of the germs on surfaces. Sanitizing is often done with a bleach-and-water solution. It can also be accomplished with high heat.

scaffold: To gradually build skills or knowledge.

secondhand smoke: Tobacco smoke inhaled by someone who is not smoking. For example, children can inhale secondhand smoke when they are in the same room or ride in a vehicle with adults who are smoking. Exposure to secondhand smoke is thought to be nearly as dangerous as smoking (www.mayoclinic.com/health/secondhand-smoke/CC00023).

sedentary: Word used to describe lifestyles or activities that involve little physical activity.

serving: The amount of food recommended by the U.S. Department of Agriculture's MyPlate. For example, one serving of milk equals one cup.

shaken baby syndrome: Also known as *abusive head trauma*. Used to describe the signs and symptoms resulting from violent shaking of an infant or small child, resulting in brain damage. The degree of brain damage depends on the amount, duration, and force of shaking.

shelter in place: A precaution used in situations in which remaining in the building is safer than evacuation. Typically sheltering in place means staying indoors. In some extreme situations additional precautions such as turning off air conditioning and fans are recommended to prevent potential exposure to airborne contamination.

simple carbohydrates: Carbohydrates that can be broken down easily by the body. While some occur naturally in healthy foods like milk and fruit, many simple carbohydrates come from nutritionally void foods like doughnuts, cookies, candy, and soda.

standard precautions: Prevention practices involving blood and blood-containing body fluids used to minimize exposure to blood-borne illnesses and infections. Standard precautions assume that all blood and blood-containing body fluid may be infected. They use barriers, such as gloves, and the cleaning and disinfecting of contaminated surfaces to prevent transmission. Standard precautions may also be referred to as *universal precautions*.

structured/planned activity: Any activity planned to meet specific learning objectives. These are often led or guided by a caregiver/teacher. For example, a caregiver may plan to dance with scarves to support children's development of coordination and rhythm.

sudden infant death syndrome, or SIDS: Unexpected and sudden death of an infant (a child under one year of age). Investigation and autopsy do not reveal explainable causes of death.

sudden unexpected infant death, or SUID: Sudden and unexplained death of an infant in which the manner and cause of death are not immediately obvious.

sympathy: Compassion for another's situation or experience.

temperament: Combination of behavioral and emotional traits or characteristics that are present at birth. These influence how a child responds to environment, people, and experiences.

thirdhand smoke: Residue remaining on hair, clothes, and other surfaces after someone smokes. For example, adults who smoke cigarettes retain hundreds of toxins on their hair and clothes. When they cuddle young children, the children can inhale the toxins into their lungs or absorb them through skin contact.

trans fat: A category of fats that are added to many foods to enhance flavor and preserve shelf life but are associated with health problems.

transition: Change from one activity, state, or place to another. Daily transitions between activities or events occur throughout the day. Other transitions occur when a child changes classrooms, programs, or caregivers or moves to an elementary school.

unstructured/unplanned activity: Any activity with no specific learning objectives, although development may occur. For example, children may play on a climber during outdoor time.

use zones: Areas immediately beneath and surrounding play equipment. These areas must contain shock-absorbing material at least twelve inches in depth to soften children's falls.

vehicle safety restraint: Equipment used so young children can ride safely in cars, vans, and buses. Vehicle safety restraints can be car seats, booster seats, or manufacturer-installed harness systems (seat belts). The type of restraint used must match the child's age and size to be safe and effective.

vigorous activity: Activity that increases a person's heart rate, makes breathing harder, and usually includes sweating.

volatile organic compounds (VOCs): Chemicals released as gases from substances such as paint. VOCs are respiratory irritants that can cause respiratory distress for some children and adults. Most VOCs produce odors, though some do not. Plastics, paints, glues, electronic equipment, and printer inks are the most common sources of VOCs.

whole grains: Grains or foods made from grains that have all the essential elements still intact and have not been processed.

References

AAFA (Asthma and Allergy Foundation of America). 2011. "Allergy Facts and Figures." Accessed February 25, 2012. www.aafa.org/display.cfm?id=9&sub=30.

AAP (American Academy of Pediatrics). 2011. "Media Use by Children Younger Than 2 Years." *Pediatrics* 128 (5): 1040–45. doi: 10.1542/peds.2011-1753.

AAP (American Academy of Pediatrics). 2012. "About Childhood Obesity." Accessed March 28, 2012. www2.aap.org/obesity/about.html.

AAP, APHA, and NRC (American Academy of Pediatrics, American Public Health Association, and National Resource Center for Health and Safety in Child Care and Early Education). 2010. "Preventing Childhood Obesity in Early Care and Education Programs." Selected Standards from *Caring for Our Children: National Health and Safety Performance Standards,* 3rd ed. http://nrckids.org/CFOC3/PDFVersion/preventing_obesity.pdf.

AAP, APHA, and NRC (American Academy of Pediatrics, American Public Health Association, and National Resource Center for Health and Safety in Child Care and Early Education). 2011. *Caring for Our Children: National Health and Safety Performance Standards; Guidelines for Early Care and Education Programs,* 3rd ed. Elk Grove Village, IL: AAP; Washington, DC: APHA.

AHA (American Heart Association). 2012. "Overweight in Children." Accessed February 6, 2012. www.heart.org/HEARTORG/GettingHealthy/Overweight-in-Children_UCM_304054_Article.jsp.

Almon, Joan, and Edward Miller. 2011. "The Crisis in Early Education: A Research-Based Case for More Play and Less Pressure." *Alliance for Childhood*, November, 1–4.

Baker, Amy C. and Lynn A. Manfredi/Petitt. 2004. *Relationships, the Heart of Quality Care: Creating Community Among Adults in Early Care Settings.* Washington, DC: National Association for the Education of Young Children.

Betancourt, Jeanette. 2012. "Healthy Habit for Life." Greenbush Healthy Living. Accessed April 2, 2012. www.gbhealthyliving.com/vnews/display.v/SEC/Teachers%7CHealthy%20Habits%20for%20Life.

Block, Gladys. 2004. "Foods Contributing to Energy Intake in the US: Data from NHANES III and NHANES 1999–2000." *Journal of Food Composition and Analysis* 17:439–47. doi:10.1016/j.jfca.2004.02.007.

Bloom, Paula Jorde, Ann Hentschel, and Jill Bella. 2010. *A Great Place to Work: Creating a Healthy Organizational Climate.* Lake Forest, IL: New Horizons.

Boise, Phil. 2010a. *Go Green Rating Scale for Early Childhood Settings.* St. Paul, MN: Redleaf Press.

Boise, Phil. 2010b. *Go Green Rating Scale for Early Childhood Settings Handbook: Improving Your Score.* St. Paul, MN: Redleaf Press.

Borse, Nagesh N., Julie Gilchrist, Ann M. Dellinger, Rose A. Rudd, Michael F. Ballesteros, and David A. Sleet. 2008. "CDC Childhood Injury Report: Patterns of Unintentional Injuries among 0–19 Year Olds in the United States, 2000–2006." Atlanta: Centers for Disease Control and Prevention; National Center for Injury Prevention and Control. www.cdc.gov/SafeChild/images/CDC-ChildhoodInjury.pdf.

Cali, Anna M. G., and Sonia Caprio. 2008. "Obesity in Children and Adolescents." *Journal of Endocrinology and Metabolism* 93 (11): S31–S36. doi:10.1210/jc.2008-1363.

CASEL (Collaborative for Academic, Social, and Emotional Learning). 2007. "Background on Social and Emotional Learning (SEL)." *CASEL briefs.* University of Illinois. http://casel.org/wp-content/uploads/2011/04/SELCASELbackground.pdf.

CDC (Centers for Disease Control and Prevention). 1997. "Guidelines for School and Community Programs to Promote Lifelong Physical Activity among Young People." www.cdc.gov/mmwr/preview/mmwrhtml/00046823.htm.

CDC (Centers for Disease Control and Prevention). 2010. "After the Baby Arrives." Last modified April 1. www.cdc.gov/ncbddd/pregnancy_gateway/after.html.

CDC (Centers for Disease Control and Prevention). 2012. "Heads Up: Prevent Shaken Baby Syndrome." Accessed February 20, 2012. www.cdc.gov/concussion/headsup/sbs.html.

CPSC (Consumer Product Safety Commission). 1999. "CPSC Staff Study of Safety Hazards in Child Care Settings." www.cpsc.gov/LIBRARY/ccstudy.html.

CPSC (Consumer Product Safety Commission). 2011. "Updated: The New Crib Standard; Questions and Answers." www.cpsc.gov/onsafety/2011/06/the-new-crib-standard-questions-and-answers.

CSSP (Center for the Study of Social Policy). 2007. *Strengthening Families: A Guidebook for Early Childhood Programs,* 2nd ed. www.cssp.org/publications/neighborhood-investment/strengthening-families/top-five/strengthening-families-a-guidebook-for-early-childhood-programs.pdf.

Donoghue, Elaine A., and Colleen A. Kraft, eds. 2010. *Managing Chronic Health Needs in Child Care and Schools: A Quick Reference Guide.* Elk Grove Village, IL: American Academy of Pediatrics.

Durlak, Joseph A., Roger P. Weissberg, Allison B. Dymnicki, Rebecca D. Taylor, and Kriston B. Schellinger. 2011. "The Impact of Enhancing Students' Social and Emotional Learning: A Meta-Analysis of School-Based Universal Interventions." *Child Development* 82 (1): 474–501. doi: 10.1111/j.1467-8624.2010.01564.x.

ERIC Clearinghouse on Elementary and Early Childhood Education. 1994. "Children's Nutrition and Learning." ERIC Digests. www.ericdigests.org/1994/nutrition.htm.

FEMA (Federal Emergency Management Agency). 2006. "Earthquake Preparedness: What Every Child Care Provider Needs to Know." www.fema.gov/library/viewRecord.do?id=1520.

Fox, Lise, Glen Dunlap, Mary Louise Hemmeter, Gail E. Joseph, and Phillip S. Strain. 2003. "The Teaching Pyramid: A Model for Supporting Social Competence and Preventing Challenging Behavior in Young Children." *Young Children* 58 (4): 48–52.

Fox, Lise, and Rochelle Harper Lentini. 2006. "'You Got It!' Teaching Social and Emotional Skills." *Young Children* 61 (6): 1–7.

Galinksy, Ellen. 2010. *Mind in the Making: The Seven Essential Life Skills Every Child Needs.* New York: HarperStudio.

Gladwell, Malcolm. 2008. *Outliers: The Story of Success.* New York: Little, Brown.

Honig, Alice Sterling. 2010. *Little Kids, Big Worries: Stress-Busting Tips for Early Childhood Classrooms.* Baltimore: Paul H. Brookes.

Jacobson, Tamar. 2008. *"Don't Get So Upset!" Help Young Children Manage Their Feelings by Understanding Your Own.* St. Paul, MN: Redleaf Press.

Kersey, Katharine C., and Marie L. Masterson. 2011. "Learn to Say Yes! When You Want to Say No! to Create Cooperation Instead of Resistance." *Young Children* 66 (4): 40–44.

KFF (The Kaiser Family Foundation). 2004. "The Role of Media in Childhood Obesity." www.kff.org/entmedia/upload/The-Role-Of-Media-in-Childhood-Obesity.pdf.

Maher, Erin J., Guanghui Li, Louise Carter, and Donna B. Johnson. 2008. "Preschool Child Care Participation and Obesity at the Start of Kindergarten." *Pediatrics* 122 (2): 322–30. doi:10.1542/peds.2007-2233.

Masten, Ann S. 2001. "Ordinary Magic: Resilience Processes in Development." *American Psychologist* 56 (3): 227–38. doi: 10.1037/0003-066X.56.3.227.

Mischel, Walter, Yuichi Shoda, and Monica L. Rodriguez. 1989. "Delay of Gratification in Children." *Science* 244 (4907): 933–38.

Mission: Readiness. 2009. "Ready, Willing, and Unable to Serve." http://cdn.missionreadiness.org/MR-Ready-Willing-Unable.pdf.

Mitchell, Anne. 2000. "The Case for Credentialing Directors Now and Considerations for the Future." In *Managing Quality in Young Children's Programs: The Leader's Role*, edited by Mary L. Culkin, 152–69. New York: Teachers College Press.

MLRC (Minnesota Learning Resource Center). 2004. "S.M.A.R.T." www.themlrc.org/about/about_programs.htm.

Mooney, Carol Garhart. 2010. *Theories of Attachment: An Introduction to Bowlby, Ainsworth, Gerber, Brazelton, Kennell, and Klaus*. St. Paul, MN: Redleaf Press.

Morgan, Gwen G. 2000. "The Director as a Key to Quality." In *Managing Quality in Young Children's Programs: The Leader's Role*, edited by Mary L. Culkin, 40–58. New York: Teachers College Press.

NAEYC (National Association for the Education of Young Children). 2008. "Teacher-Child Ratios within Group Size." www.naeyc.org/files/academy/file/Teacher-Child_Ratio_Chart_9_16_08.pdf.

National Center on Shaken Baby Syndrome. 2011. "All about SBS/AHT." Accessed June 19, 2012. http://dontshake.org/sbs.php?topNavID=3&subNavID=317.

National Research Council and Institute of Medicine. 2000. *From Neurons to Neighborhoods: The Science of Early Childhood Development*. Edited by Jack P. Shonkoff and Deborah A. Phillips. Washington, D.C.: National Academy Press.

National Scientific Council on the Developing Child and National Forum on Early Childhood Policy and Programs. 2010. "The Foundations of Lifelong Health Are Built in Early Childhood." Center on the Developing Child at Harvard University. http://developingchild.harvard.edu/index.php/download_file/-/view/700/.

Nitzke, Susan, Dave Riley, Ann Ramminger, and Georgine Jacobs. 2010. Rethinking Nutrition: Connecting Science and Practice in Early Childhood Settings. St. Paul: Redleaf Press.

Nord, Mark, Alisha Coleman-Jensen, Margaret Andrews, and Steven Carlson. 2010. *Household Food Security in the United States, 2009*. Economic Research Report, 108. US Department of Agriculture. www.ers.usda.gov/Publications/ERR108/ERR108.pdf.

Ogden, Cynthia, and Margaret Carroll. 2010. "Prevalence of Obesity among Children and Adolescents: United States, Trends 1963–1965 through 2007–2008." Centers for Disease Control and Prevention. www.cdc.gov/nchs/data/hestat/obesity_child_07_08/obesity_child_07_08.htm.

Sedlak, Andrea J., Jane Mettenburg, Monica Basena, Ian Petta, Karla McPherson, Angela Green, and Spencer Li. 2010. "Fourth National Incidence Study of Child Abuse and Neglect (NIS-4): Report to Congress." US Department of Health and Human Services; Administration for Children and Families; Office of Planning, Research, and Evaluation; and the Children's Bureau. www.acf.hhs.gov/programs/opre/abuse_neglect/natl_incid/index.html.

Seith, David, and Elizabeth Isakson. 2011. *Who Are America's Poor Children? Examining Health Disparities Among Children in the United States*. National Center for Children in Poverty. http://nccp.org/publications/pub_995.html.

Sesame Street Child Resilience Initiative. 2011. "Sesame Street Child Resilience Initiative: Developing Resilience Factors." Accessed October 28, 2012. www.sesameworkshop.org/what-we-do/our-work/finding-strength-in-the-face-of=adversity-32-detail.html.

Shaping America's Youth. 2012. "The Skyrocketing Cost of Obesity: It's Everybody's Business." Accessed April 2, 2012. www.shapingamericasyouth.org/Skyrocketing%20Costs%20of%20Obesity-032510.pdf?cid=328.

Shapiro-Mendoza, Carrie. 2012. "Sudden, Unexplained Infant Death Investigation: A Systematic Training Program for the Professional Infant Death Investigation Specialist." Centers for Disease Control and Prevention. www.cdc.gov/sids/TrainingMaterial.htm#manual.

Shenk, Joshua Wolf. 2009. "What Makes Us Happy?" *The Atlantic*, June. www.theatlantic.com/magazine/archive/2009/06/what-makes-us-happy/7439/.

Stern, Robin. 2012. "Social and Emotional Learning: What Is It? How Can We Use It to Help Our Children?" NYU Child Study Center. Accessed February 2, 2012. www.aboutourkids.org/articles/social_emotional_learning_what_it_how_can_we_use_it_help_our_children.

Task Force on Sudden Infant Death Syndrome. 2011. "SIDS and Other Sleep-Related Infant Deaths: Expansion of Recommendations for a Safe Infant Sleeping Environment." *Pediatrics* (October): 1030–39. doi:10.1542/peds.2011-2284.

US HHS, CDC, and PCPFS (United States Department of Health and Human Services, Centers for Disease Control and Prevention, and the President's Council on Physical Fitness and Sports). 1996. *Physical Activity and Health: A Report of the Surgeon General Executive Summary.* www.cdc.gov/NCCDPHP/SGR/pdf/execsumm.pdf.

USDA (United States Department of Agriculture). 1999. *Healthy Eating Helps You Make the Grade!* www.fns.usda.gov/tn/Resources/makethegrade.pdf.

WhiteHouse.gov. 2010. "Child Nutrition Reauthorization Healthy, Hunger-Free Kids Act of 2010." www.whitehouse.gov/sites/default/files/Child_Nutrition_Fact_Sheet_12_10_10.pdf.

White House Task Force on Childhood Obesity. 2010. *Solving the Problem of Childhood Obesity within a Generation, Report to the President.* www.letsmove.gov/sites/letsmove.gov/files/TaskForce_on_Childhood_Obesity_May2010_FullReport.pdf.

Why Hunger. 2012. "U.S. Hunger: Statistics on Federal Food Programs." WhyHunger.org. Accessed April 2, 2010. www.whyhunger.org/frontend.php/overlay/simpleIndex?id=2055.

Willis, Clarissa A., and Pam Schiller. 2011. "Preschoolers' Social Skills Steer Life Success." *Young Children* 66 (1): 42–48.

Index

Certificate
of Participation

Our program is pursuing the recommendations put forth in

Healthy Children, Healthy Lives

The Wellness Guide for Early Childhood Programs

to ensure that we support and enhance

children's health and wellness. Ask us how!

Participating program

Sharon Bergen, PhD

Rachel Robertson, MA

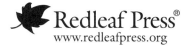

Redleaf Press®
www.redleafpress.org

Seven complete PowerPoint presentations!

You're using **Healthy Children, Healthy Lives** to integrate wellness throughout your program. Now, use **Healthy Children, Healthy Lives Training and Resources** to present the program to staff members, stakeholders, and families.

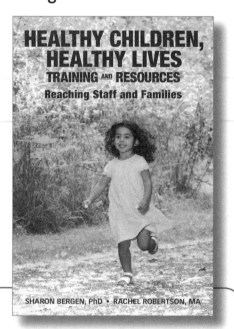

This CD-ROM contains everything you need to explain the many ways that *Healthy Children, Healthy Lives* can improve your program and bring wellness to each person that passes through the doors.

INCLUDES

Seven PowerPoint presentations

- An overview of the *Healthy Children, Healthy Lives* program for families and stakeholders
- Six comprehensive trainings to present the content and application of the wellness guide to staff members

Printable files

- Family resource flyers focusing on a broad range of wellness topics
- Resource flyers for staff members focusing on how wellness topics relate to their daily work
- Handouts for each PowerPoint presentation

Visit www.RedleafPress.org or call 800-423-8309 to order now.

HEALTHY CHILDREN, HEALTHY LIVES TRAINING AND RESOURCES

Sharon Bergen, PhD
Rachel Robertson, MA

CD-ROM   Product #541648-BR

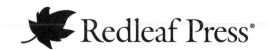